The Doctor Sebi Diet: The Complete Guide to a Plant-Based Diet

77 Simple, Doctor Sebi Alkaline Diet Recipes & Food List for Weight Loss, Liver Cleansing, Removing Phlegm & Mucus

OLIVIA SHIELDS

DEDICATION

This book is dedicated to people who want to live a healthy life!

Copyright © 2020 Olivia Shields

All rights reserved.

No part of this book may be reproduced in any form or by any electronic or mechanical means – except in the case of brief quotation embodied in articles or reviews – without written permission from its publisher.

ISBN: 9781653818747

DISCLAIMER

The information and recipes contained in this book are provided for acquaintance only. Please, consult with a qualified healthcare provider before making any changes in your diet or lifestyle. The author does not assume any liability or responsibility to use all or any information contained in this book to anyone with respect to any loss or damage caused or alleged to be caused directly or indirectly from the provided information.

All images are from stock.adobe.com.

CONTENTS

Introduction 8

The Doctor Sebi Diet 10
    What is the Doctor Sebi Diet? 10
    Food Principles 12
    The Doctor Sebi Diet and Weight Loss 14
    Benefits and Downsides 15
    Doctor Sebi's Supplements 17
    Reverse Disease 20

Doctor Sebi's Food List 22
    Approved Products 22
        Vegetable List 23
        Fruit List 24
        Grain List 25
        Spices and Seasonings 25
        Teas, Oil, Nuts and Seeds 26
    Products to Avoid 28

Doctor Sebi Inspired Recipes 29
    Soups 29
        Creamy Cucumber Gazpacho 30
        Vegetable Soup/Broth 32
        Mushroom Soup 34
        Spicy Tomato Bean Soup 36
        Vegan Clam Chowder 38
    Salads 41
        Sautéed Kale 42
        Wakame Salad 44
        Strawberry Dandelion Salad 46
        Healthy Salad 48
        Grilled Romaine Lettuce 50
        Rainbow Salad 52
        Everyday Salad 54
    Main Dishes 56
        Jamaican Jerk Patties 57
        Zucchini Bread Pancakes 60

Basil Avocado Pasta 62
Kamut Patties 64
Portobello Mushroom Burgers 66
Creamy Kamut Pasta 69
Macaroni and Cheese 72
Healthy Fried-Rice 74
Meatballs 76
Zucchini Noodles with Avocado Sauce 78
Vegetarian Fajitas 80
Homemade Hummus 82
Zucchini Hummus Wrap 84
Sausage Links 86
Garbanzo Bean Burger 88
Margherita Pizza 91
Ravioli 94
Chickpea French Fries 98
Homemade Pasta 100
Vegetarian Lasagna 102
Kamut Cereal 106
Vegan "Ribs" 108
Stuffed Bell Peppers 110

Sauces **113**
Sweet Barbecue Sauce 114
Avocado Sauce 116
Fragrant Tomato Sauce 118
"Cheese" Sauce 120
Guacamole 122
"Garlic" Sauce 124

Special Ingredients **126**
Spicy Infused Oil 127
Homemade Walnut Milk 128
"Garlic" Infused Oil 129
Aquafaba 130
Homemade Hempseed Milk 132
Papaya Seed Mango Dressing 134
Tomato Ginger Dressing 136
Dill Cucumber Dressing 138

    Italian Infused Oil 140
Snacks & Bread **142**
    Onion Rings 143
    Flatbread... 146
    Healthy Crackers 148
    Tortillas.. 150
    Tortilla Chips 152
Desserts **154**
    Squash Pie.. 155
    Strawberry Sorbet... 158
    Blueberry Muffins 160
    Banana Strawberry Ice Cream 162
    Homemade Whipped Cream.. 164
    "Chocolate" Pudding 166
    Banana Nut Muffins 168
    Mango Nut Cheesecake 170
    Blackberry Jam 172
    Blackberry Bars... 174
Smoothies **176**
    Creamy Mango Smoothie 177
    Fluffy Avocado Pear Smoothie 178
    Apple Pie Smoothie 180
    Morning Energizer Smoothie... 182
    Sunshine Smoothie 184
    Green Detox Smoothie 186
    Vegan Detox Smoothie.. 188
    Mixed Berry Smoothie 190
    Hydrating Recovery Smoothie 192
    Immune Booster Smoothie 194
    Sweet and Tart Smoothie 196
    Berry Peach Smoothie 198
Conclusion **200**

SPECIAL GIFT FOR YOU

Thank you for buying my book!

Sign up for my newsletter to receive free or discounted Kindle books.

After you have joined my newsletter, you will receive a notification when my books are available to download for FREE on Amazon, no charge.

You will also receive messages when I publish a new book and they will be available to you with a big discount.

As promised, I want to provide you with a shopping list of approved Doctor Sebi products for FREE. It will help prevent you from buying unnecessary products.

This file will be sent to your email in PDF format and can be opened on your phone, tablet or laptop.

Just follow this link or scan QR Code to sign up and receive your shopping list!

http://bit.ly/Sebi2020

You will definitely love it!

Thank you for staying with me!

INTRODUCTION

Alfredo Darrington Bowman, well known as Doctor Sebi, was a Honduran herbalist, pathologist, naturalist, and biochemist. He studied and observed different herbs in Africa, South and Central America, the Caribbean, and North America. Based on his 30 years of experience, he developed a unique methodology for curing the human body with herbs and a specialized diet.

This diet was called the Doctor Sebi Diet. It is a plant-based diet that consists of a short list of approved foods and a long list of additional supplements. The Doctor Sebi Diet is not the easiest diet, however it has helped many ailing people feel better without taking pills.

Doctor Sebi developed this diet for those who wish to naturally prevent or cure disease and improve their health without relying on standard Western medicine.

In this book, you will find information about the Doctor Sebi Diet and its food principles, a list of approved products and herbs, and 77 simple recipes that you can cook quickly for you and your family.

Specifically, in the next sections, you will learn:

- What the Doctor Sebi Diet is?

- How it works?
- Main principles of the diet.
- Approved list of products and herbs.
- Benefits and downsides of the Doctor Sebi Diet.
- How to reverse disease following this diet?
- How to lose weight on the diet?

77 easy recipes for soups, salads, main dishes, desserts, smoothies, sauces, snacks, and breads based on Doctor Sebi's approved food list.

Ready to read further?

Let's go...

THE DOCTOR SEBI DIET

WHAT IS THE DOCTOR SEBI DIET?

The Doctor Sebi Diet was developed by Alfredo Darrington Bowman, a self-taught herbalist who found excellent nutritional value in some foods. Despite his name, however, Doctor Sebi did not hold a Ph.D., nor was he a medical practitioner.

He claimed these plant-based meals had the potential to help people prevent diseases, and they could serve as treatment plans for chronic medical conditions such as diabetes.

This diet is composed of greens, vegetables, and other plants which are intended to create alkaline conditions in the body.

Doctor Sebi explained that high acidity levels promote pathogen development and create an environment that fosters the creation of disease-causing mucus. For instance, pneumonia is caused by mucus accumulation in the lungs, while diabetes is a result of excess mucus in the pancreas.

According to Sebi, his diet raises the alkaline level in your body. This in turn prevents the formation of mucus and makes it difficult for infection-causing organisms to survive.

Furthermore, this diet induces cell rejuvenation and the elimination of toxic substances from the blood and body, promoting improved health and stronger resistance to illnesses.

There are many Doctor Sebi approved supplements that, combined with the recommended foods, constitute this diet.

Bowman designed this nutrition plan for people who wish to use natural methods to prevent or treat their medical conditions. It was aimed at minimizing reliance on Western medicine and relying more on holistic approaches to bettering your health.

For an in-depth analysis of what constitutes this popular diet, we are going to look closer at the details in the subsequent sections. This will include the types of foods to eat, the benefits and drawbacks of the diet, its significance to weight loss, the supplements involved, and how it reverses medical illnesses.

FOOD PRINCIPLES

There are strict food rules that need to be followed to gain optimal results from Doctor Sebi's diet. You will have to make it a routine to adhere to the program for an indefinite amount of time, it is a lifelong endeavor. Bowman claimed that for the body to continually heal itself you will have to continually eat the listed foods.

You should know that this program is entirely plant-based, a vegan diet. It consists of nuts and seeds, grains, fruits, vegetables, herbs, and oils. Consuming animal products is wholly prohibited.

The rules surrounding this diet are stringent. They hinge on keeping individuals away from processed foods and animal products, while encouraging them to take the listed supplements. These rules are not scientifically grounded nutritional guidelines.

There are eight rules to follow:

1. You are only allowed to eat the foods listed in the nutritional guide.

2. You are supposed to drink 3.8 liters of water (1 gallon) every day.

3. Doctor Sebi's supplements are to be consumed an

hour before taking any medication.

4. Animal products (including meat, milk, eggs, etc.) are not allowed.

5. Alcohol consumption is not permitted.

6. Do not consume wheat products at all. You are only supposed to eat "natural growing grains" that are outlined in the nutritional guide.

7. Use of microwaves is not permitted as it is considered to kill the nutrients present in foods.

8. Canned and seedless fruits are prohibited.

From the descriptions above, you'll notice that the diet is devoid of proteins. This is because aside from banning animal products (that are a rich source of protein), it also forbids soy products, lentils, and some beans.

But, if you want to consume plant-based proteins, you can complete the nutritional needs for the diet and gain the most out of it. It's only your choice. Protein makes up an integral part of your diet since it helps in muscle development, the formation of hair and nails, and healthy skin and joints.

THE DOCTOR SEBI DIET AND WEIGHT LOSS

While it is not designed for weight loss, this diet can ultimately help you shed some extra pounds. It discourages the consumption of ultra-processed foods and other Western diets that can be high in fat and sugar.

People who stick to plant-based diets for the most part have lower bodyweight and fewer cases of congenital medical conditions.

Moreover, most of the foods eaten with this program have a low-caloric content, aside from the oils, avocados, nuts, and seeds. Although this diet may help you lose weight, it does not guarantee that you will maintain your new weight once you resume your previous eating patterns. Studies have shown that most people end up gaining weight again once they stop following the Sebi diet. Perhaps reiterate the point that the diet is intended to be followed for life.

The absence of calorie valuation with each recipe and supplement also makes it challenging to gauge the sustainability of weight loss on the diet.

BENEFITS AND DOWNSIDES

The benefits:

1. One of the most significant benefits of Doctor Sebi's diet is its promotion of consuming of fruits and vegetables. These two food categories have high fiber content, antioxidants, and many essential minerals and vitamins.

2. The diet contains many plant compounds that have been known to combat inflammation and improve immunity against a myriad of illnesses.

3. Studies done by scientists and other experts have shown that people who consume fruits and vegetables in high amounts every day have a reduced risk and fewer incidents of cardiovascular diseases and cancer.

4. This diet is rich in fibers, especially from whole grains and vegetables. Fibers are beneficial in that they help deal with constipation and ease bowel movements.

5. Limiting ultra-processed foods improves the quality of the diet in the overall scheme of things.

The downsides:

1. It is highly restrictive. Doctor Sebi's diet forbids many foods, including all animal products. This restriction extends to some types of fruits, tomatoes, vegetables, etc. Such

limitations may cause a person to develop a negative relationship with food.

2. The diet also encourages a reliance on supplements that are not intended to be substituted for foods with caloric value. Real food should always be your primary source of nutrients.

3. It lacks essential nutrients such as proteins that are necessary for the healthy development of the body. To meet your daily quota while relying solely on the listed foods for protein, you would have to consume large quantities of them every day. Lack of essential proteins can affect hormone and enzyme production, muscle development, and skin structure.

4. The diet is not based on scientific evidence. There are many claims surrounding Doctor Sebi's diet. However, none of them have been scientifically proven thus far.

DOCTOR SEBI'S SUPPLEMENTS

In addition to eating the foods listed in Doctor Sebi's nutritional guide, you will also be required to buy his proprietary supplements. Bowman guaranteed they would aid in cleansing your body and nourishing your cells.

The recommended package is the all-inclusive option, consisting of all 20 of the available supplements. This is said to be the best option because it is the fastest means of cleansing and restoring the body.

Alternatively, you can opt to purchase individual supplements based on your health goals. Each has its unique benefits. For more details, let's take a look at some of the supplements and what they offer.

1. **Green Food Plus** – This supplement contains multiple minerals collected from herbs that are rich in chlorophyll. It promotes the healthy development of vital organs such as the brain, nervous system, heart, and the blood. You should take 4 capsules each day.

2. **Viento** – A cleanser and an energizer, Viento will revitalize your body and increase the oxygen levels in your brain and blood. It is rich in iron, which is used in the formation of hemoglobin in red blood cells. The supplement

also works on your kidneys and the lymphatic, respiratory, and central nervous systems. You should consume 4 capsules per day.

3. **Sea Moss/Seaweed** – This nutritious plant is a rich source of calcium, magnesium, iron, and ninety-two other essential minerals. It also contains many vitamins and is quite versatile in how you can ingest it. Sea moss can be incorporated in baking, blended into smoothies, used as an ingredient for gravies, ice creams, and fashioned into desserts. It is well known for its healing aspects and ability to promote a balanced restoration of the mucous membrane, thus improving your overall health. The ailments it can help treat include skin conditions, respiratory diseases, and muscle and joint pains.

4. **Testo** – It works on your endocrine system. It promotes hormonal balance and improves your libido and virility, especially in men. Some claims suggest it helps increase blood flow to male genitalia, which enhances sexual responsiveness.

5. **Tooth Powder** – Just as its name suggests, it nourishes the teeth and cleanses your gums while preventing dental diseases such as tooth decay. The powder is applied to a wet toothbrush.

6. **Uterine Wash and Oil** – This wash restores the health of the vaginal canal.

7. **Estro** – This product promotes fertility and high

libido in women. The dosage is 4 capsules every day.

8. **Hair Follicle Fortifier** – For hair growth and strengthened hair follicles, make a paste and apply it evenly on your scalp every day.

9. **Banju** – It handles conditions involving the nervous system such as stress, pain, and irritability. There is also a tonic version that caters to children with ADHD and ADD. Consume 2 tablespoons twice a day.

Other available supplements include:
- Bromide Plus Powder.
- Eva Salve for skin nourishment.
- Bio Ferro capsules for blood purification.
- Eyewash for cleansing the eyes.
- Iron Plus for fighting inflammation.
- Hair Food Oil for scalp and hair nourishment.

Something worth noting is that these supplements do not provide a guide on all the nutrients contained in them and in what quantities. This, therefore, makes it difficult to know if by taking them you will meet your daily nutritional requirements.

REVERSE DISEASE

The question of whether Doctor Sebi's diet can reverse diseases is one that still sparks debate today. Alfredo Bowman championed his cause that the diet could provide relief to people with various ailments. Among others these include diabetes, heart conditions, liver problems, herpes, and kidney issues.

His premise suggested that the foods altered your body's pH and made it more alkaline, thus aiding in fighting disease. Science, however, says otherwise. According to research, foods can alter the alkalinity level of your urine, but they do not affect the blood's pH.

However, this does not mean that all is lost. On the contrary, this diet has many health and medical benefits.

Fruits and vegetables improve heart function and strengthen it. This makes the heart capable of combating disease and reduces the risk of heart attacks.

Because the diet is low in fat, it also serves as an excellent way to prevent atherosclerosis and the accumulation of fatty deposits in your blood vessels. Healthy blood vessels allow proper blood flow and minimize strain on your heart.

Your body will also get a healthy balance of

macronutrients and vitamins from the listed foods. This fosters an overall improvement in health.

Rich in fiber, this diet can help persons suffering from constipation cope with the condition and even reverse it. Seeds, vegetables, fruits, and nuts all play critical roles in easing bowel movements.

Doctor Sebi's diet has many health benefits, but it comes with several drawbacks. Fortunately, there is a way around them. By consuming plant-based protein sources such as beans and lentils, you can complete the nutritional needs for a well-rounded diet and gain the most benefit. If you suffer from any chronic condition or you are taking certain medications, consult your doctor before transitioning to this diet.

DOCTOR SEBI'S FOOD LIST

APPROVED PRODUCTS

Doctor Sebi strongly believed that people should strictly eat only non-GMO foods. This approved list of products includes vegetables and fruits which are not seedless or otherwise altered, and they contain many minerals and vitamins that occur naturally.

While the vegetable list is extensive, the list of fruits is much smaller as many types of fruits should be avoided according to Doctor Sebi. The herbs list is the shortest, as it is difficult to find herbs that have remained unaltered.

However, in its entirety, this prepared Doctor Sebi Food List is long and diverse. It contains a variety of options to create a wide array of delicious dishes.

Vegetable List

Vegetables	
Amaranth Greens (Callaloo, a variety of greens)	Wild Arugula
Avocado	Bell Peppers
Chayote (Mexican Squash)	Cucumber
Dandelion Greens	Garbanzo Beans
Izote (Cactus flower, Cactus leaf)	Kale
Lettuce (all types, except Iceberg)	Mushrooms (all types, except Shitake)
Nopales (Mexican Cactus)	Okra
Olives	Onions
Sea Vegetables (Wakame, Arame, Hijiki, Dulse, Nori)	Squash
Tomato (Cherry and Plum only)	Tomatillo
Turnip Greens	Zucchini
Watercress	Purslane (Verdolaga)

Fruit List

Fruits	
Apples	Bananas (Baby or Burro only)
Berries (all, except Cranberries)	Cantaloupe
Cherries	Currants
Dates	Figs
Grapes (seeded only)	Limes (Key Limes preferred, with seeds)
Mango	Melons (seeded only)
Orange (Seville or sour preferred)	Papayas
Peaches	Pears
Plums	Prickly Pear (Cactus Fruit)
Prunes	Raisins (seeded only)
Soft Jelly Coconuts	Soursop (West Indian or Latin markets)
Tamarind	

Grain List

Grains	
Amaranth	Fonio
Kamut	Quinoa
Rye	Spelt
Tef	Wild Rice

Spices and Seasonings

Mild Flavors	
Basil	Bay Leaf
Cloves	Dill
Oregano	Savory
Sweet Basil	Tarragon
Thyme	

Sweet Flavors	
Pure Agave Syrup (from cactus)	Date Sugar

Pungent & Spice Flavors	
Achiote	Cayenne Pepper
African Bird Pepper	Onion Powder
Habanero	Sage

Salty Flavors	
Pure Sea Salt	Powdered Granulated Seaweed (Kelp, Dulce, Nori – have a "sea taste")

Sweet Flavors	
Pure Agave Syrup (from cactus)	Date Sugar

Teas, Oil, Nuts and Seeds

Herbal Teas	
Burdock	Chamomile
Elderberry	Fennel
Ginger	Raspberry
Tila	

Oils	
Olive Oil (Do not cook)	Coconut Oil (Do not cook)
Grape Seed Oil	Hempseed Oil
Avocado Oil	Sesame Oil

Nuts & Seeds	
Hemp seeds	Raw Sesame Seeds
Raw Sesame "Tahini" Butter	Walnuts
Brazil Nuts	

PRODUCTS TO AVOID

Any food that is not included in the list of approved Doctor Sebi's products is not permitted, for example:

- eggs,
- fish,
- seedless fruits,
- canned vegetables or fruits,
- red meat,
- wheat,
- alcohol,
- sugar (except agave syrup and date sugar),
- dairy,
- poultry,
- fortified foods,
- foods made with baking powder,
- processed foods,
- restaurant or take-out foods,
- yeast,
- and soy products.

Moreover, many fruits, vegetables, seeds, nuts, and grains are not allowed according to the diet. Only foods from the approved list may be eaten.

DOCTOR SEBI INSPIRED RECIPES
SOUPS

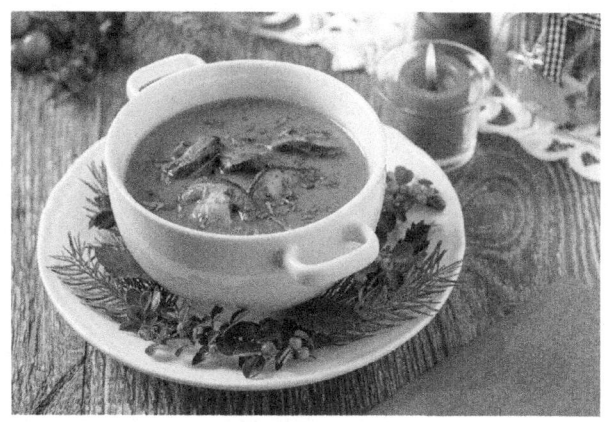

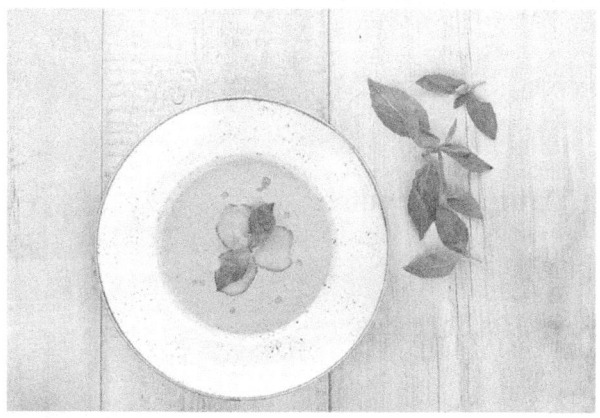

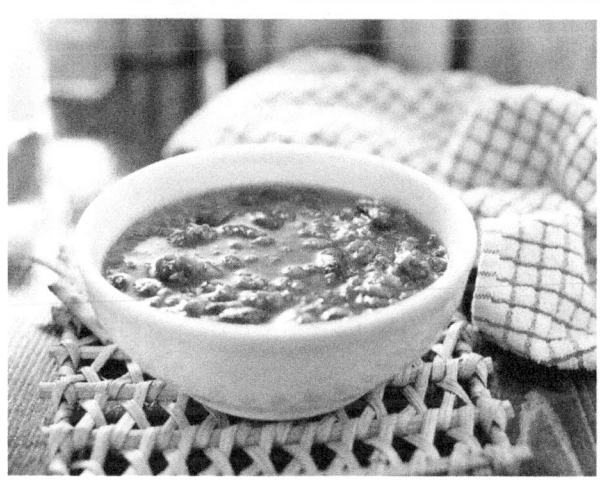

Creamy Cucumber Gazpacho

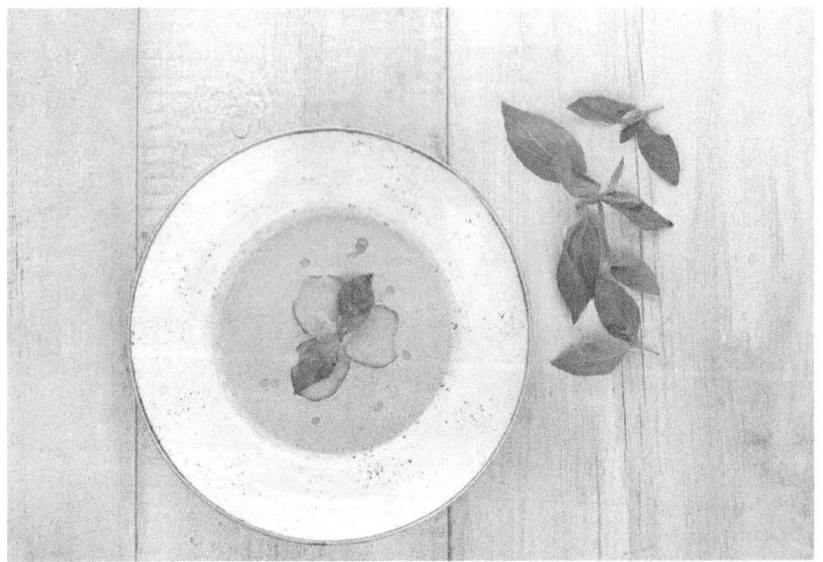

Cooking Time: 15 Minutes

Serving Size: 2 Servings

Ingredients

- 1 ripe Avocado
- 2 handfuls of Basil
- 1 Cucumber
- juice from 1 Key Lime
- 1 1/4 teaspoons of Pure Sea Salt
- 2 cups of Spring Water

Cooking Instructions

1. Store all ingredients, except Pure Sea Salt, in a refrigerator until cold.
2. Peel the Cucumber and remove seeds.
3. Add all ingredients to a blender and puree until smooth with some green specks.
4. Pour the mixture into a pot with a lid.
5. Put the soup back in the refrigerator. Allow it to chill.
6. Serve and garnish with basil leaves and thinly sliced Cucumber.
7. Enjoy your Creamy Cucumber Gazpacho!

Vegetable Soup/Broth

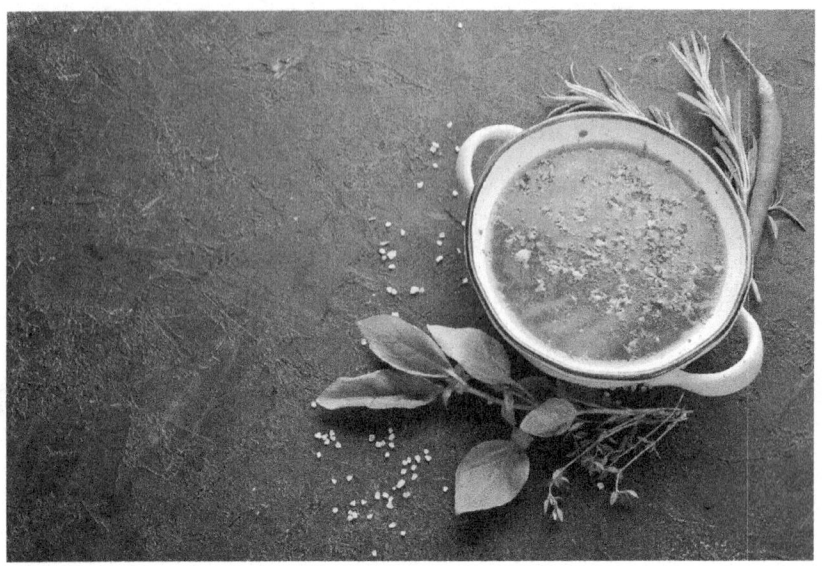

Cooking Time: 1 Hour 20 Minutes

Serving Size: 5-6 Servings

Ingredients

- 1 cup of sliced Bell Peppers
- 2 chopped Plum Tomatoes
- 1 1/2 cups of chopped Mushrooms
- 1 cup of chopped Kale
- 1 cup of sliced White and Red Onions
- 1/2 cup of mashed Green Onions
- 2 cups of chopped Butternut Squash
- 4 cups of *Aquafaba (see recipe on page 130)*
- 1 teaspoon of Onion Powder
- 1/2 teaspoon of Cayenne Powder**

- 1 teaspoon of Dill
- 1 teaspoon of Oregano
- 1 teaspoon of Basil
- 1 teaspoon of Savory
- 1 teaspoon of Sage
- 1 teaspoon of Pure Sea Salt
- 1 tablespoon of Grape Seed Oil
- 4 cups of Spring Water

Cooking Instructions

1. Add Mushrooms, Onions, Peppers and Grape Seed Oil to a stockpot. Sauté vegetables on medium heat for about 5 minutes.
2. Add Spring Water and *Aquafaba*.
3. Add all other vegetables and seasonings to the pot. Bring the mixture to a rolling boil.
4. Reduce to low heat and cook for 1 to 2 hours.
5. Serve and enjoy your Vegetable Soup!

Useful Tips

*If you don't have prepared *Aquafaba*, simply add 4 more cups of Spring Water.

**If you prefer less spice, omit Cayenne Powder or add only 1/4 teaspoon instead.

If you want to make Vegetable Broth, let it cool, strain the vegetables out, and serve it.

Mushroom Soup

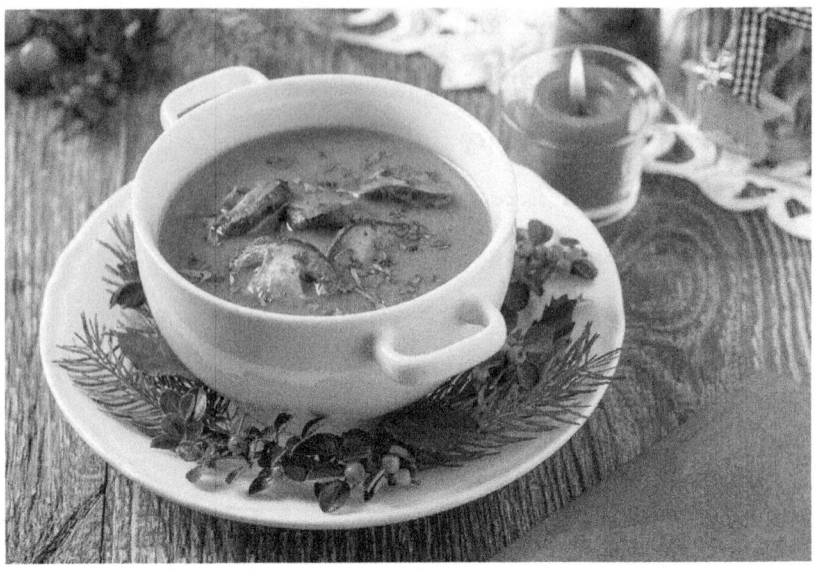

Cooking Time: 45 Minutes

Serving Size: 6-8 Servings

Ingredients
- 3 cups of sliced Mushrooms
- 1 1/2 cups of Garbanzo Bean Flour
- 1 cup of mashed Onions
- 2 cups of chopped Chayote Squash
- 1 cup of *Homemade Hempseed Milk (see recipe on page 132)**
- 1 cup of *Aquafaba (see recipe on page 130)**
- 1 tablespoon of Onion Powder
- 1 teaspoon of Cayenne Powder

- 2 teaspoons of Basil
- 2 teaspoons of Pure Sea Salt
- 1-2 tablespoons of Grape Seed Oil
- 6 cups of Spring Water

Cooking Instructions

1. Peel the Chayote Squash and cut it into cubes.
2. Add Grape Seed Oil, Mushrooms, and Onions to a large pot. Sauté vegetables on medium heat for 4 to 5 minutes.
3. Pour 4 cups of Spring Water, *Aquafaba*, and *Homemade Hempseed Milk*.
4. Add Chayote Squash and seasonings to the pot, stir and bring to a boil.
5. Put Garbanzo Bean Flour and 2 cups of Spring Water into a blender and blend thoroughly for about 30 seconds until there are no lumps.
6. Add the prepared mixture to the stockpot and cook on low heat for about 30 minutes. Stir occasionally.
7. Serve** and enjoy your Mushroom Soup!

Useful Tips

*If you don't have prepared *Aquafaba*, use *Vegetable Broth* instead *(see recipe on page 32)*. If you have neither, add one more cup of Spring Water.

**You can serve this soup with our *Healthy Crackers* *(see recipe on page 148)*.

Spicy Tomato Bean Soup

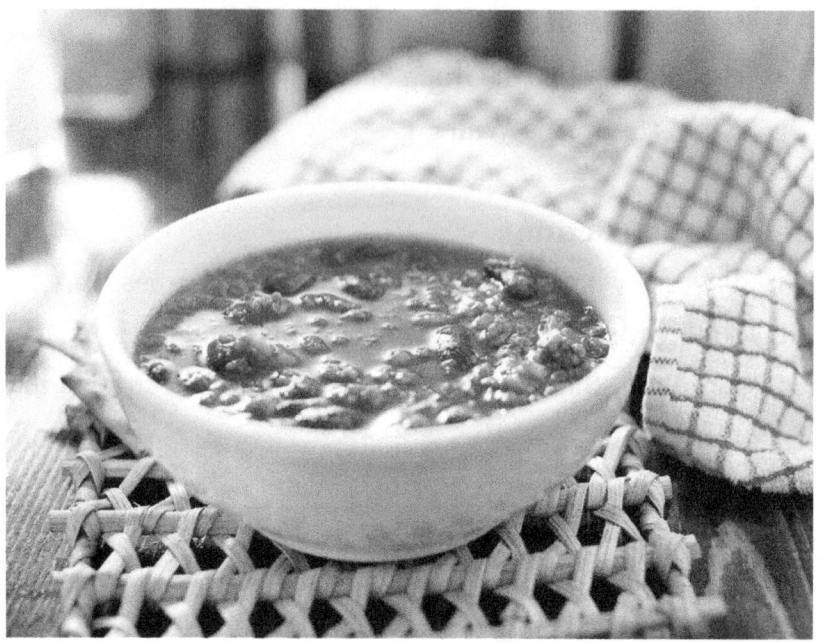

Cooking Time: 1 Hour 20 Minutes

Serving Size: 6-8 Servings

Ingredients

- 10 chopped Plum Tomatoes
- 1 chopped Tomatillo
- 3 cups of cooked Garbanzo Beans
- 1/2 cup of chopped Red Bell Pepper
- 1/2 cup of minced Onions
- 1/2 cup of chopped Green Bell Pepper
- 2 teaspoons of Onion Powder

- 1 teaspoon of Cayenne Powder*
- 1 teaspoon of Sweet Basil
- 1 teaspoon of Oregano
- 1/2 teaspoon of Achiote
- 2 teaspoons of Pure Sea Salt
- 2 teaspoons of Grape Seed Oil
- 1 cup of Spring Water
- Prepared *Sausage Links (see recipe on page 86)*

Cooking Instructions

1. Add Grape Seed Oil, Bell Peppers, Onions and Tomatillo to a large pot.
2. Sauté vegetables on medium heat for 4 to 5 minutes.
3. Put Garbanzo Beans, seasonings, Tomatoes, and Spring Water to the stockpot.
4. Stir and bring to a boil.
5. Cook on low heat for about 1 hour. Stir occasionally.
6. Cut the *Sausage Links* into slices and add them a couple of minutes before the soup is fully cooked.
7. Serve and enjoy your Spicy Tomato Soup!

Useful Tips

*If you prefer less spice, add only 1/2 teaspoon of Cayenne instead.

Vegan Clam Chowder

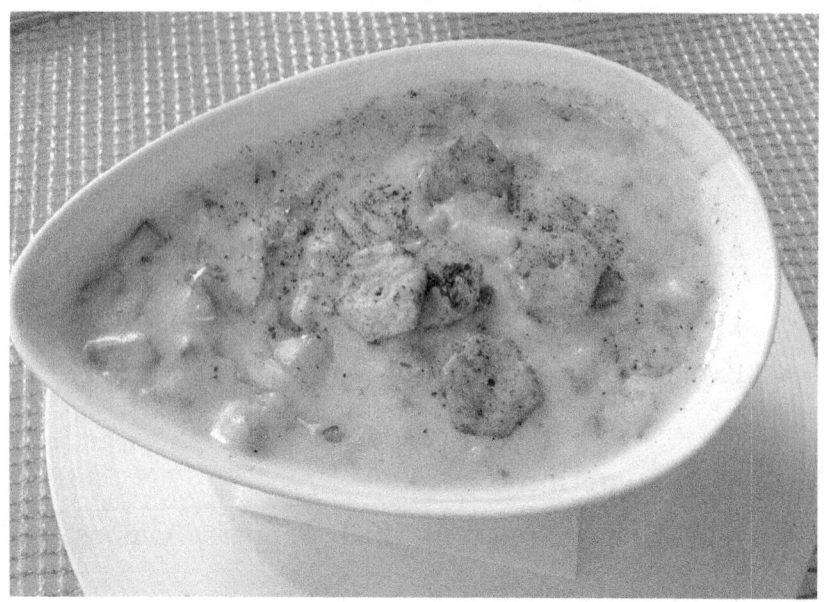

Cooking Time: 40 Minutes

Serving Size: 6-8 Servings

Ingredients

- 1 1/2 cups of cooked Garbanzo Beans
- 1 1/2 cups of chopped Oyster Mushrooms*
- 2 cups of Garbanzo Bean Flour
- 1 cup of mashed White Onions
- 1/2 cup of chopped Butternut Squash
- 1/2 cup of medium diced Kale
- 1 cup of *Homemade Hempseed Milk (see recipe on page 132)***

- 1 cup of *Aquafaba (see recipe on page 130)****
- 2 teaspoons of Dill
- 1/2 teaspoon of Cayenne Powder
- 2 teaspoons of Basil
- 1 tablespoon of Pure Sea Salt
- 1 tablespoon of Grape Seed Oil
- 7 cups of Spring Water

Cooking Instructions

1. Pour *Aquafaba* and 6 cups of Spring Water into a large pot.
2. Add cooked Garbanzo Beans, chopped vegetables, and half of each seasoning to the pot.
3. Bring to a rolling boil and cook on medium heat for 10 minutes, stirring occasionally.
4. Whisk *Hempseed Milk*, Grape Seed Oil, 1 cup of Spring Water and the rest of the seasonings in a separate bowl. Slowly whisk in the Chickpea Flour.
5. Continue adding the flour, whisking constantly, until it is fully combined and there are no lumps.
6. Slowly pour the mixture into the pot with vegetables and whisk to avoid lumps.
7. Add chopped Oyster Mushrooms and cook on low heat for 10 minutes. Stir the soup occasionally.
8. Serve**** and enjoy your Vegan Clam Chowder!

Useful Tips

*If you don't have Oyster Mushrooms you may use any mushrooms you have on hand. However, Oyster Mushrooms are the best alternative to clams.

**If you don't have *Homemade Hempseed Milk,* you can substitute *Homemade Walnut Milk (see recipe on page 128).*

***If you don't have prepared *Aquafaba,* use *Vegetable Broth* instead *(see recipe on page 32).* If you have neither, substitute one additional cup of Spring Water.

****You can serve this Vegan Clam Chowder Soup with our *Healthy Crackers (see recipe on page 148).*

SALADS

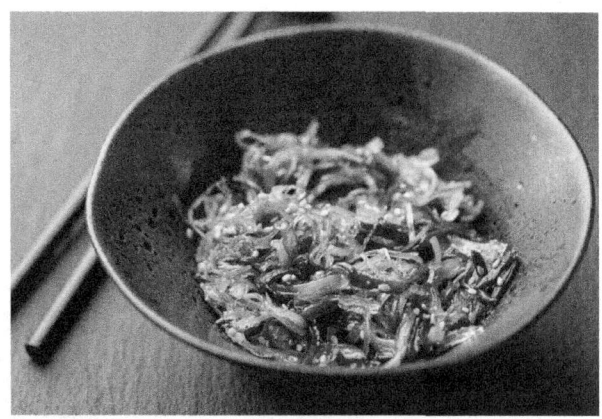

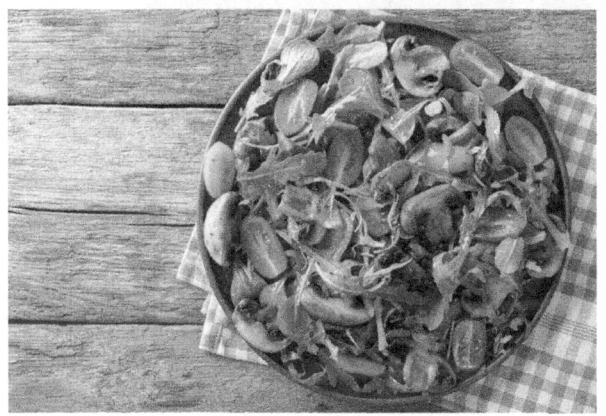

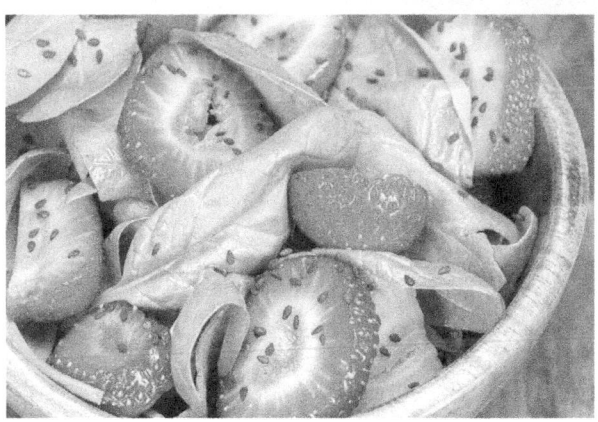

Sautéed Kale

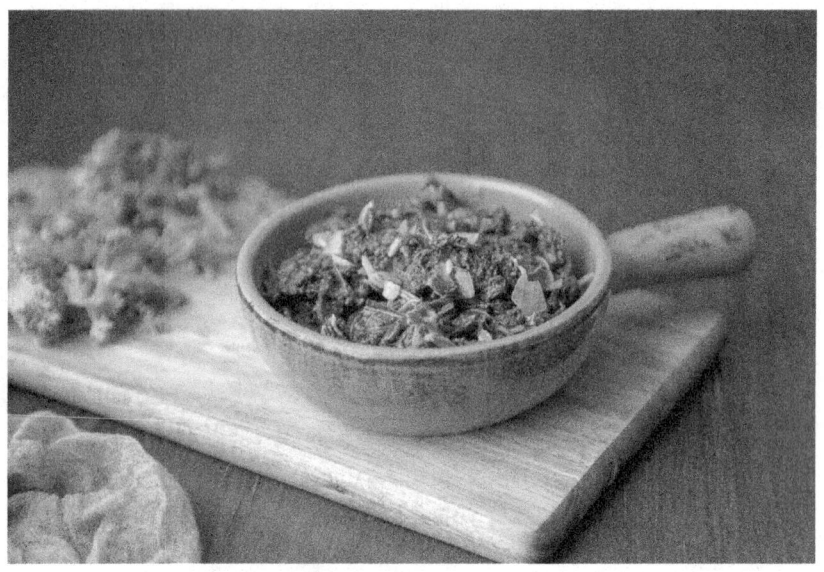

Cooking Time: 15 Minutes

Serving Size: 4 Servings

Ingredients

- 1 bunch of Kale
- 1/4 cup of minced Red Pepper
- 1/4 cup of minced Onions
- 2 tablespoons of *"Garlic" Infused Oil (see recipe on page 129)*
- 1/4 teaspoon of Pure Sea Salt
- 1 teaspoon of Crushed Red Pepper flakes

Cooking Instructions

1. Fold rinsed Kale leaves in half and cut off the stems.
2. Dice Kale into small pieces. Spin in a salad spinner** until dry.
3. Warm a wok on high heat and pour in *"Garlic" Infused Oil.**
4. Add minced Peppers and Onions to the wok and sauté on medium heat for 2 to 3 minutes.
5. Add Kale leaves and Pure Sea Salt to the pan and cover with a lid. Reduce to low heat and cook for about 5 minutes.
6. Spread crushed Red Pepper flakes and mix thoroughly. Cover with a lid and continue cooking for 3 minutes.
7. Serve and enjoy your Sautéed Kale Salad!

Useful Tips

* If you don't have *"Garlic" Infused Oil* prepared, substitute Grape Seed Oil instead.

** If you don't have a salad spinner, wait until the Kale is dry to continue.

Wakame Salad

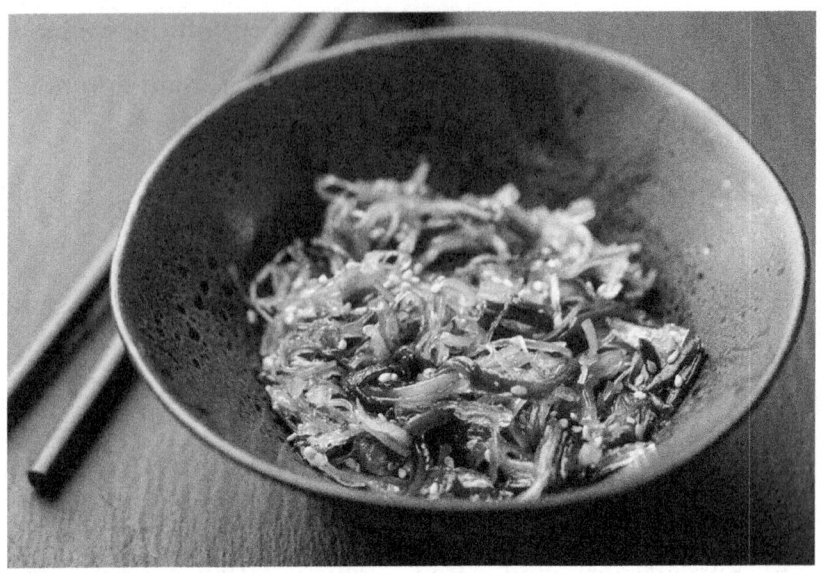

Cooking Time: 15 Minutes

Serving Size: 2 Servings

Ingredients

- 2 cups of Wakame Stems
- 1 tablespoon of Sesame Seeds
- 2 tablespoons of diced Red Bell Pepper
- 1 teaspoon of Ginger
- 1 tablespoon of Agave Syrup
- 1 teaspoon of Onion Powder
- 1 tablespoon of Sesame Oil

- 1 tablespoon of Key Lime juice
- Spring Water for soaking

Cooking Instructions

1. Put Wakame Stems in a medium bowl and cover them with Spring Water.
2. Soak Wakame stems for 8 to 10 minutes until soft then drain the water.
3. In a separate bowl, combine Agave Syrup, Onion Powder, Sesame Oil, Ginger and Key Lime juice and whisk them thoroughly.
4. Place diced Bell Pepper and soaked Wakame on a plate. Pour dressing over the salad.
5. Sprinkle Sesame Seeds on top.
6. Enjoy your Wakame Salad!

Strawberry Dandelion Salad

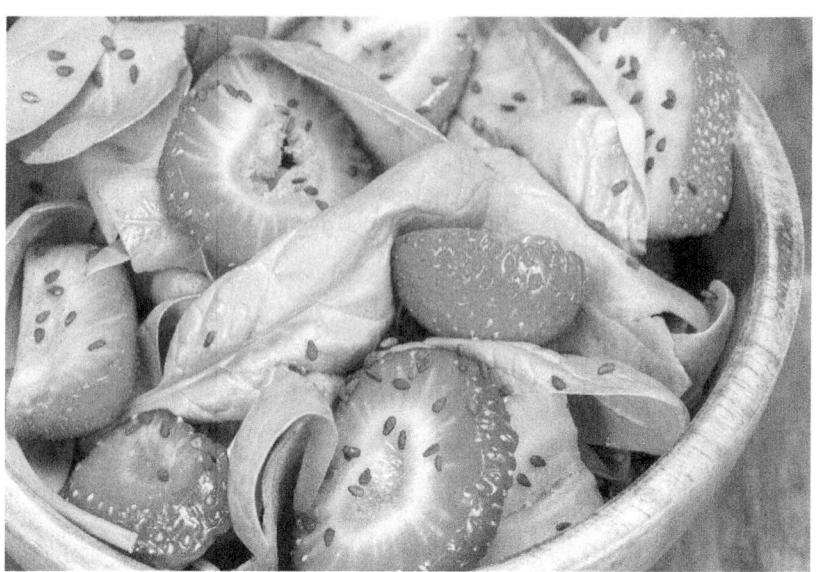

Cooking Time: 10 Minutes

Serving Size: 2 Servings

Ingredients

- 10 sliced Strawberries
- 4 cups of Dandelion Greens
- 1 sliced Red Onion
- 1 tablespoon of Sesame Seeds
- 2 tablespoons of Key Lime juice
- 2 tablespoons of Grape Seed Oil
- Pure Sea Salt, to taste

Cooking Instructions

1. Add Grape Seed oil to a non-stick frying pan and warm it on medium heat.
2. Sprinkle Pure Sea Salt on the Red Onions and put the slices in the warm pan.
3. Sauté until Onions are slightly golden and soft. Stir often.
4. Before Onions are fully cooked, add 1 teaspoon of Key Lime Juice and continue cooking for 1 to 2 minutes.
5. In a salad bowl, mix 1 teaspoon of Key Lime Juice with sliced Strawberries.
6. Wash the Dandelion Greens, tear them into medium pieces, and add to the bowl.
7. Add cooked Onions with their Juice into the salad bowl.
8. Sprinkle Sesame Seeds and Pure Sea Salt on top.
9. Enjoy your Strawberry Dandelion Salad!

Healthy Salad

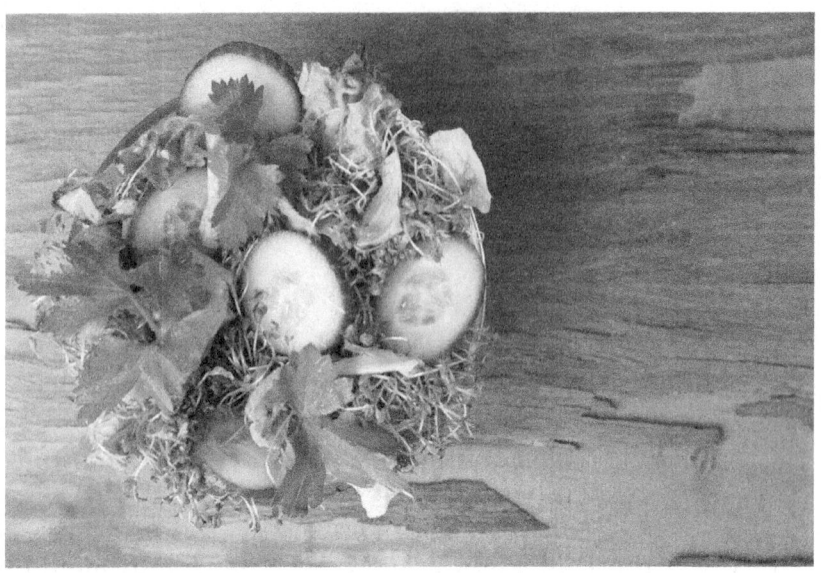

Cooking Time: 5 Minutes

Serving Size: 2 Servings

Ingredients

- 2 cups of torn Watercress
- 1/2 of sliced Cucumber
- 1 tablespoon of Key Lime Juice
- 2 tablespoons of Olive Oil
- Pure Sea Salt, to taste
- Cayenne Powder, to taste

Cooking Instructions

1. Pour Key Lime Juice and Olive Oil into a salad bowl. Mix them well to combine.
2. Slice the Cucumber and add to the bowl.
3. Tear Watercress and add to the bowl.
4. Sprinkle Cayenne Powder and Pure Sea Salt on top according to your liking.
5. Mix thoroughly.
6. Enjoy your quick Detox Salad!

Grilled Romaine Lettuce

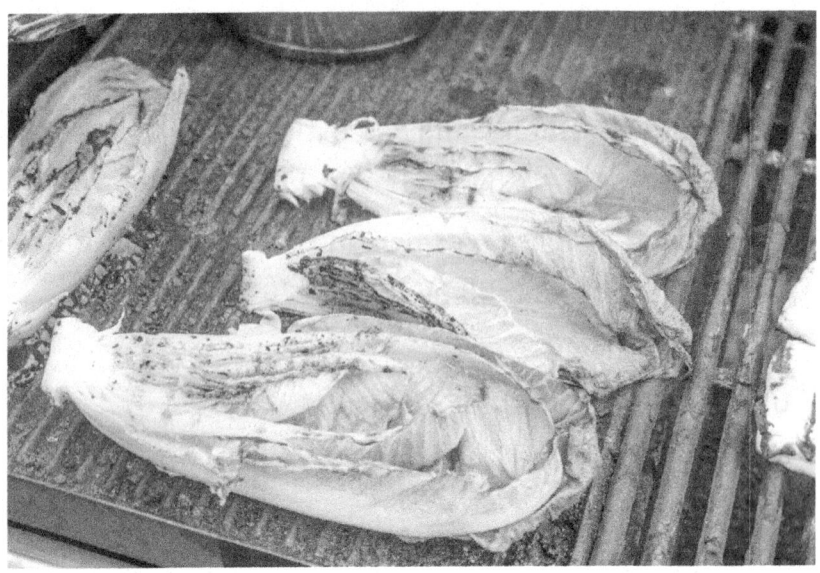

Cooking Time: 15 Minutes

Serving Size: 2 Servings

Ingredients

- 4 heads of Romaine Lettuce
- 1 tablespoon of minced fresh Basil
- 1 tablespoon of diced Red Onion
- 1 tablespoon of Agave Syrup
- 1 tablespoon of Key Lime Juice
- 4 tablespoons of Olive Oil
- Pure Sea Salt, to taste

- Cayenne Powder, to taste
- Onion Powder, to taste

Cooking Instructions

1. Rinse Romaine Heads and cut them in half.
2. Place Lettuce head halves on a grill. If you don't have a grill, fry them on medium heat in a large nonstick pan. Don't use any oil while cooking.
3. Grill Lettuce heads until they are browned on both sides.
4. Take cooked Romaine Lettuce off the heat and allow it to cool before serving.
5. Prepare the dressing. Combine fresh Basil, Olive Oil, Key Lime Juice, Red Onion, Agave Syrup, Pure Sea Salt, and Cayenne Powder to a small bowl. Mix thoroughly.
6. Place grilled Romaine Lettuce on a large serving plate and spoon the dressing over the salad.
7. Enjoy your Grilled Romaine Lettuce Salad!

Rainbow Salad

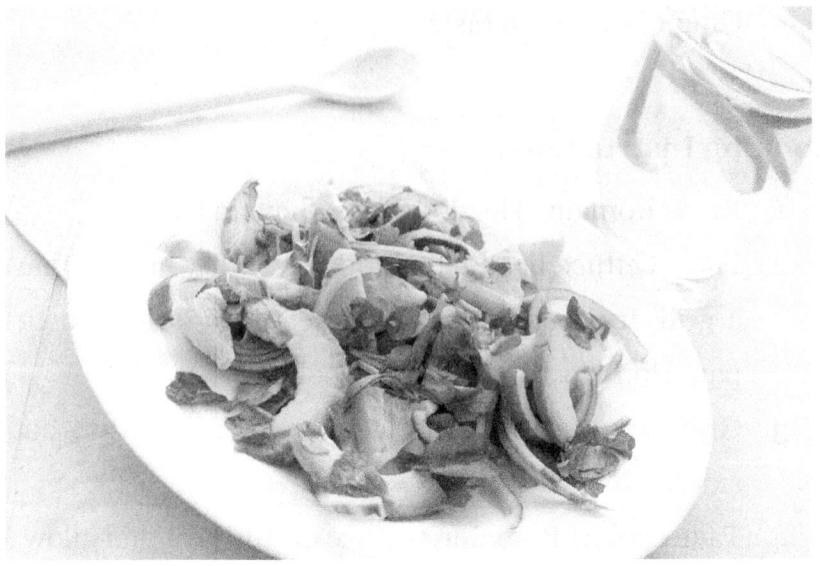

Cooking Time: 10 Minutes

Serving Size: 2 Servings

Ingredients

- 4 cups of torn Watercress
- 1 sliced Avocado
- 2 thin sliced Red Onions
- 1 chopped Seville Orange
- 2 tablespoons of Key Lime Juice
- 2 teaspoons of Agave Syrup
- 1/8 teaspoon of Pure Sea Salt
- Cayenne Powder, to taste

- 2 tablespoons of Olive Oil

Cooking Instructions

1. Prepare the Avocado. Cut it in half, peel, remove the seed, and slice.
2. Peel the Seville Orange and cut it into medium cubes.
3. Remove the skin from Red Onions and thinly slice.
4. Put Onions, Avocado, Oranges and Watercress in a salad bowl.
5. Combine Olive Oil, Cayenne Powder, Pure Sea Salt, Key Lime Juice and Agave Syrup together in a separate bowl, mix well.
6. Pour dressing on the top of the salad.
7. Enjoy your delicious Rainbow Salad!

Everyday Salad

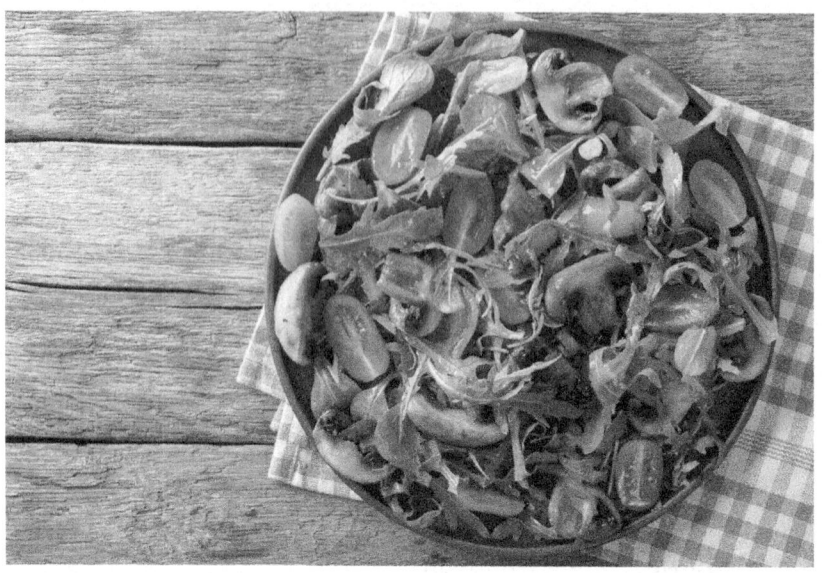

Cooking Time: 10 Minutes

Serving Size: 2 Servings

Ingredients

- 5 halved Mushrooms
- 6 halved Cherry (Plum) Tomatoes
- 6 rinsed Lettuce Leaves
- 10 Olives
- 1/2 chopped Cucumber
- juice from 1/2 Key Lime
- 1 teaspoon of Olive Oil
- Pure Sea Salt, to taste

Cooking Instructions

1. Tear rinsed Lettuce Leaves into medium pieces and put them in a medium salad bowl.
2. Add Mushroom halves, chopped Cucumber, Olives and Cherry Tomato halves into the bowl.
3. Mix well.
4. Pour Olive Oil and Key Lime juice over the salad.
5. Add Pure Sea Salt to taste. Mix it all till it is well combined.
6. Enjoy your easy Everyday Salad!

MAIN DISHES

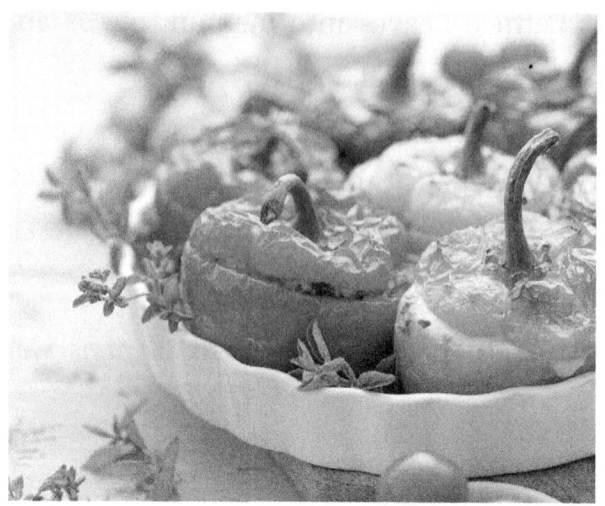

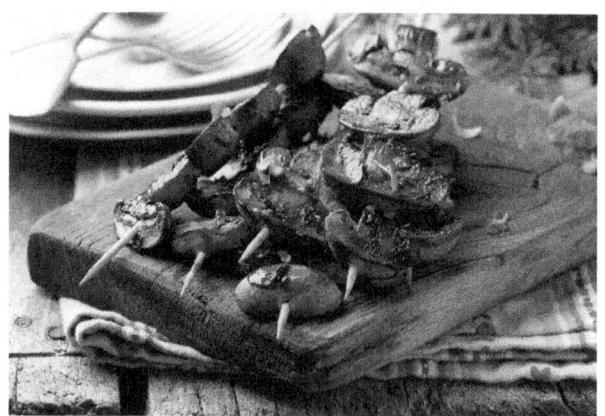

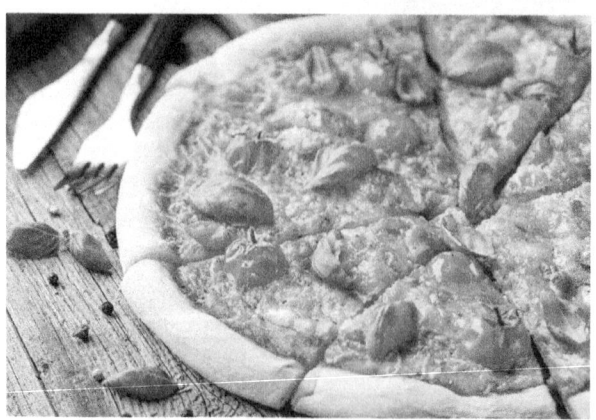

Jamaican Jerk Patties

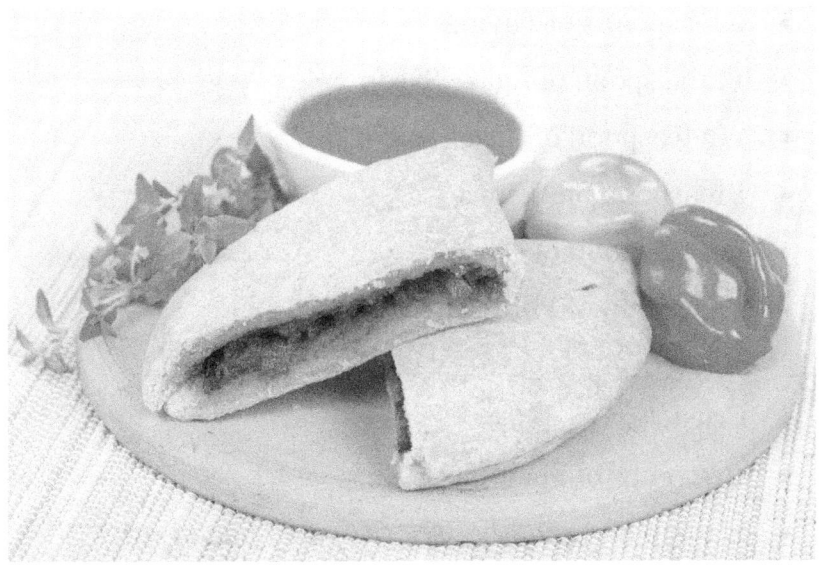

Cooking Time: 1 Hour

Serving Size: 3-4 Servings

Ingredients

Filling:
- 1 cup of cooked Garbanzo Beans
- 1/2 cup of diced Green Pepper
- 1 chopped Plum Tomato
- 2 cups of chopped Mushrooms
- 1 cup of chopped Butternut Squash
- 1/2 cup of diced Onions
- 1 tablespoon of Onion Powder

- 1 teaspoon of Ginger
- 2 teaspoons of Thyme
- 1 tablespoon of Agave Syrup
- 1/2 teaspoon of Cayenne Powder
- 1 teaspoon of Allspice
- 1/4 teaspoon of Cloves
- 1 teaspoon of Pure Sea Salt

Crust:
- 1 1/2 cups of Spelt Flour
- 1/4 cup of *Aquafaba (see recipe on page 130)*
- 1 teaspoon of Pure Sea Salt
- 1/8 teaspoon of Ginger Powder
- 1 teaspoon of Onion Powder
- 1 tablespoon of Grape Seed Oil
- 1 cup of Spring Water

Cooking Instructions

1. Preheat your oven to 350 degrees Fahrenheit.
2. Add all vegetables, excluding Cherry Tomatoes, to a food processor. Pulse a few times to chop them into large pieces.
3. Mix blended vegetables with seasonings and tomatoes in a large bowl. This constitutes the filling for the patties.

4. In a separate large bowl, combine the Spelt Flour, Grape Seed Oil and seasonings.
5. Pour in 1/2 cup of Spring Water and knead the dough into a ball, adding more water or flour as needed.
6. Leave the dough to rest for 5 to 10 minutes. Knead again for a few minutes then divide it into 8 equal parts.
7. Make each part into a ball and roll each ball out into a 6 to 7-inch circle.
8. Take a dough circle and place 1/2 cup of the filling in the center. Brush all edges of the dough with *Aquafaba*, fold it over in half and seal the edges together with a fork.
9. Repeat step 8 until all the dough circles are filled.
10. Lightly coat a baking sheet with a little Grape Seed Oil.
11. Bake filled patties for about 25 to 30 minutes until golden brown.
12. Serve* and enjoy your Jamaican Jerk Patties!

Useful Tips

*You can serve Jamaican Jerk Patties with our *Fragrant Tomato* Sauce *(see recipe on page 118)*.

Zucchini Bread Pancakes

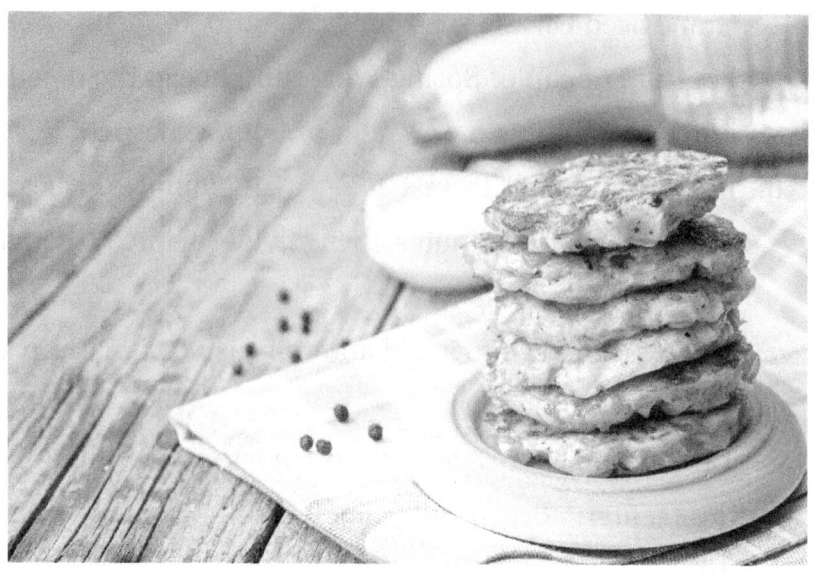

Cooking Time: 40 Minutes

Serving Size: 4 Servings

Ingredients

- 1 cup of minced Zucchini
- 2 cups of Spelt Flour*
- 1/4 cup of pureed Burro Bananas
- 1/2 cup of chopped Walnuts
- 2 tablespoons of Date Sugar
- 1 tablespoon of Grape Seed Oil
- 2 cups of *Homemade Walnut Milk (see recipe on page 128)*

Cooking Instructions

1. Take a large bowl, add Spelt Flour* and Date Sugar to it. Whisk all well.
2. Put pureed Burro Bananas and *Homemade Walnut Milk* into the bowl. Stir the mixture thoroughly until all ingredients are combined and there are no lumps.
3. Mix chopped Walnuts and minced Zucchini with other ingredients in the bowl.
4. Warm a skillet pan with Grape Seed Oil on medium heat.
5. Pour prepared some zucchini batter into the pan to form the pancakes (3 to 4 inches across).
6. Cook each pancake for about 5 minutes on each side.
7. Serve** and enjoy your Zucchini Bread Pancakes!

Useful Tips

* If you don't have Spelt Flour, you may use Kamut Flour instead.

** You can serve pancakes with Agave Syrup or our *Blackberry Jam (see recipe on page 172).*

Basil Avocado Pasta

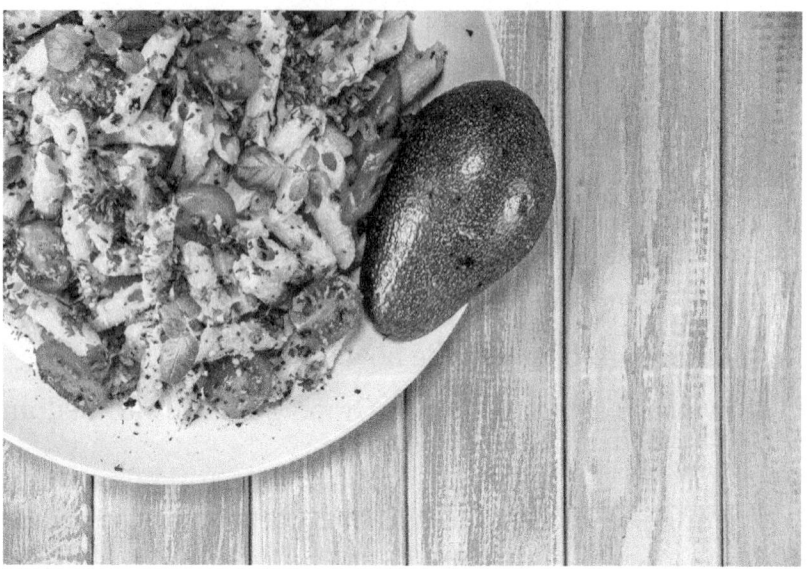

Cooking Time: 20 Minutes

Serving Size: 4 Servings

Ingredients

- 4 cups of cooked Spelt pasta
- 1 medium diced Avocado
- 2 cups of halved Cherry Tomatoes
- 1 minced fresh Basil
- 1 teaspoon of Agave Syrup
- 1 tablespoon of Key Lime Juice
- 1/4 cup of Olive Oil

Cooking Instructions

1. Place the cooked pasta in a large bowl.
2. Add diced Avocado, halved Cherry Tomatoes, and minced Basil into the bowl.
3. Stir all the ingredients until well combined.
4. Whisk Agave Syrup, Olive Oil, Pure Sea Salt and Key Lime juice in a separate bowl.
5. Pour it over the pasta and stir until well combined.
6. Enjoy your Basil Avocado Pasta!

Kamut Patties

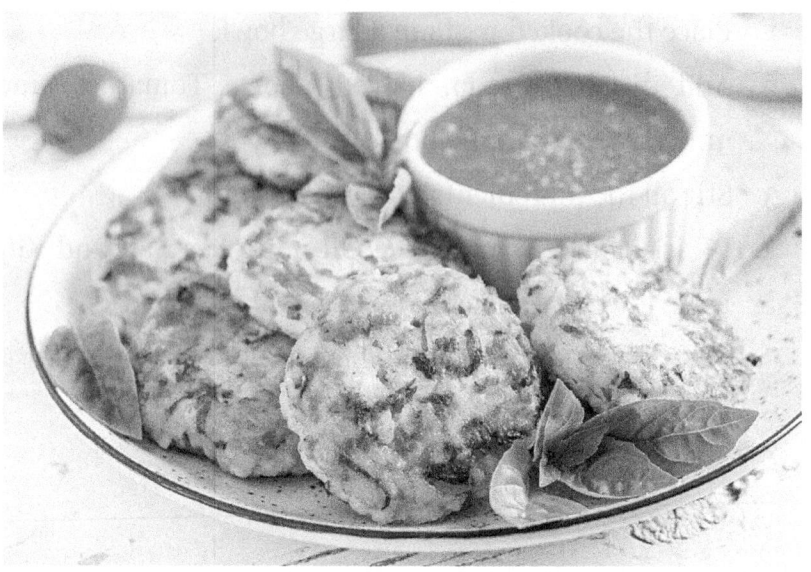

Cooking Time: 30 Minutes

Serving Size: 3-4 Servings

Ingredients

- 3 cups of cooked Kamut Cereal
- 1 cup of minced Red Onions
- 1 cup of chopped Yellow & Green Peppers
- 1 cup of Spelt Flour*
- 1/2 cup of *Homemade Hempseed Milk (see recipe on page 132)*
- 1 tablespoon of Basil

- 1/2 teaspoon of Cayenne Powder
- 1 tablespoon of Oregano
- 1 tablespoon of Onion Powder
- 1 teaspoon of Pure Sea Salt
- 2 tablespoons of Grade Seed Oil

Cooking Instructions

1. Combine vegetables, *Hempseed Milk*, seasonings, and Kamut Cereal in a large bowl.
2. Put 1/2 cup of Spelt Flour in the bowl and mix it well. Continue adding more flour until it can be formed into patties.
3. Warm Grape Seed Oil in a skillet on medium heat. Form patties from the mixture and place them on the pan.
4. Cook patties for about 4 to 5 minutes on each side.
5. Serve** and enjoy your Kamut Patties!

Useful Tips

* If you don't have Spelt Flour, add Garbanzo Bean Flour instead.

** You can serve Kamut Patties with our *"Cheese" Sauce (see recipe on page 120)* or *Fragrant Tomato Sauce (see recipe on page 118)*.

Olivia Shields

Portobello Mushroom Burgers

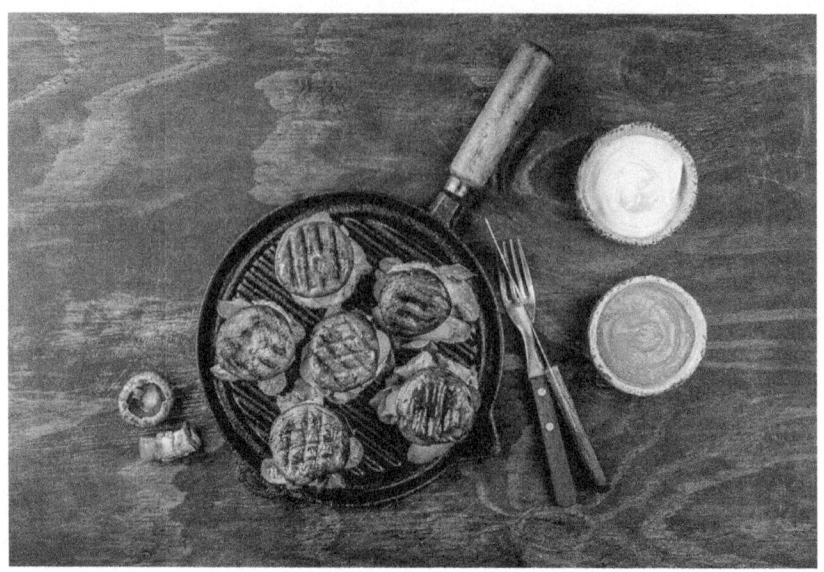

Cooking Time: 50 Minutes

Serving Size: 2 Servings

Ingredients

- 2 cups of Portobello Mushroom Caps
- 1 sliced Avocado
- 1 sliced Plum Tomatoes
- 1 cup of torn Lettuce*
- 1 cup of Purslane
- 1/2 teaspoon of Cayenne
- 1 teaspoon of Oregano

- 2 teaspoons of Basil
- 3 tablespoons of Olive Oil

Cooking Instructions

1. Preheat your oven to 425 degrees Fahrenheit.
2. Remove the mushroom stems and cut off ½ inch slice from the top slice, as if slicing a bun.
3. Mix Onion Powder, Cayenne, Oregano, Olive Oil and Basil thoroughly in a medium bowl.
4. Cover a baking sheet with foil and brush with Grape Seed Oil to avoid sticking.
5. Put mushroom caps on the baking sheet and brush them with the prepared marinade. Marinate for 10 minutes before cooking.
6. Bake for 10 minutes until golden brown then flip. Continue baking for 10 more minutes.
7. Lay out the mushroom cap on a serving dish. This will serve as the bottom for the Mushroom Burger. On it layer the sliced Avocado, Tomatoes, Lettuce, and Purslane.
8. Cover the burger with another mushroom cap. Repeat steps 7 and 8 with the remaining mushrooms and vegetables.
9. Serve** and enjoy your Portobello Mushroom Burgers!

Useful Tips

* You can add any Lettuce, except Iceberg, according to your liking.

** You can serve Portobello Mushroom Burgers with our *"Cheese" Sauce (see recipe on page 120)* or *Fragrant Tomato Sauce (see recipe on page 118)*.

Creamy Kamut Pasta

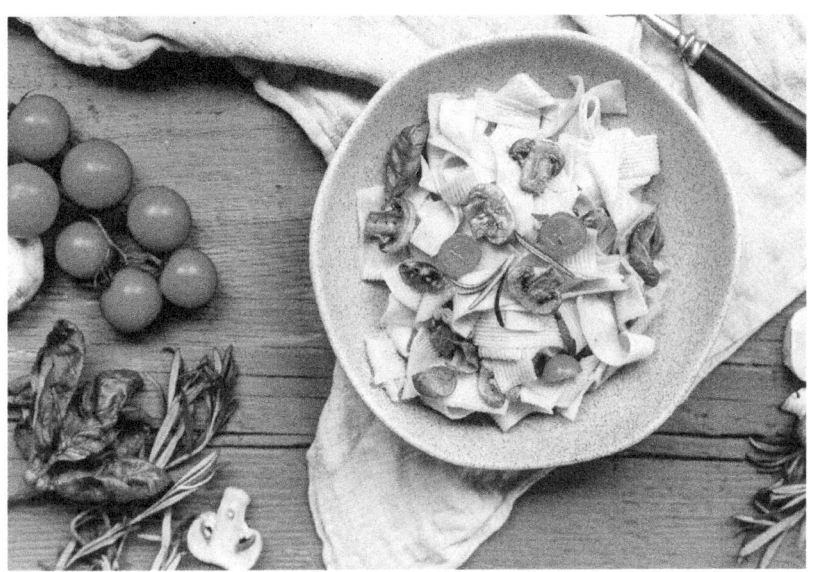

Cooking Time: 50 Minutes

Serving Size: 6 Servings

Ingredients

Pasta:

- 12 ounces of Kamut Spaghetti
- 1 tablespoon of Tarragon
- 1 teaspoon of Onion Powder
- 1 teaspoon of Pure Sea Salt
- 2 tablespoons of Grape Seed Oil
- 6 to 8 cups of Spring Water (for boiling the pasta)

Sauce:

- 2 cups of chopped Kale
- 12 chopped Cherry Tomatoes
- 1/2 diced Onion
- 2 cups of sliced Mushrooms
- 1/4 cup of Garbanzo Bean Flour
- 2 teaspoons of Onion Powder
- 1 tablespoon of Oregano
- 1 teaspoon of Tarragon
- 1 teaspoon of Basil
- 1/4 teaspoon of Pure Sea Salt + extra 1/2 teaspoon
- 1/8 teaspoon of Cayenne Powder + extra 1/8 teaspoon
- 2 tablespoons of Grape Seed Oil
- 2 cups of Coconut Milk
- 2 cups of Spring Water

Cooking Instructions

Pasta:

1. In a large pot, bring the Spring Water to a boil. Add Pure Sea Salt to taste.
2. Add Kamut Spaghetti to the boiling water. Cook for about 8 to 10 minutes until spaghetti is al dente'.
3. Drain the pasta and put it in a bowl. Add Pure Sea Salt, Tarragon, Onion Powder and Grape Seed Oil to maximize flavor.

4. Mix seasonings with pasta thoroughly.

   Sauce:

5. Add 1 tablespoon of Grape Seed Oil to a medium pot. Warm on medium heat.
6. Add sliced Mushrooms and diced Onions to the hot oil. Cook for 3 to 5 minutes, stirring occasionally.
7. Sprinkle 1/4 teaspoon of Pure Sea Salt and 1/8 teaspoon of Cayenne over the vegetables and stir.
8. Put Garbanzo Bean Flour and another tablespoon of Grape Seed Oil in the pot. Stir until it is well combined with no lumps of dry flour.
9. Add Coconut Milk, Spring Water, 1/2 teaspoon of Pure Sea Salt, Onion Powder, Oregano, Tarragon, and Basil and stir.
10. Cook on low heat for 20 minutes until it thickens slightly.
11. Add cooked pasta, chopped Tomatoes and Kale to the pot. Simmer for 3 to 5 minutes until Kale is cooked then remove from heat.
12. Serve and enjoy your Creamy Kamut Pasta!

Useful Tips

Don't store at room temperature!

Creamy Kamut Pasta can be kept in the refrigerator for 3-4 days.

Macaroni and Cheese

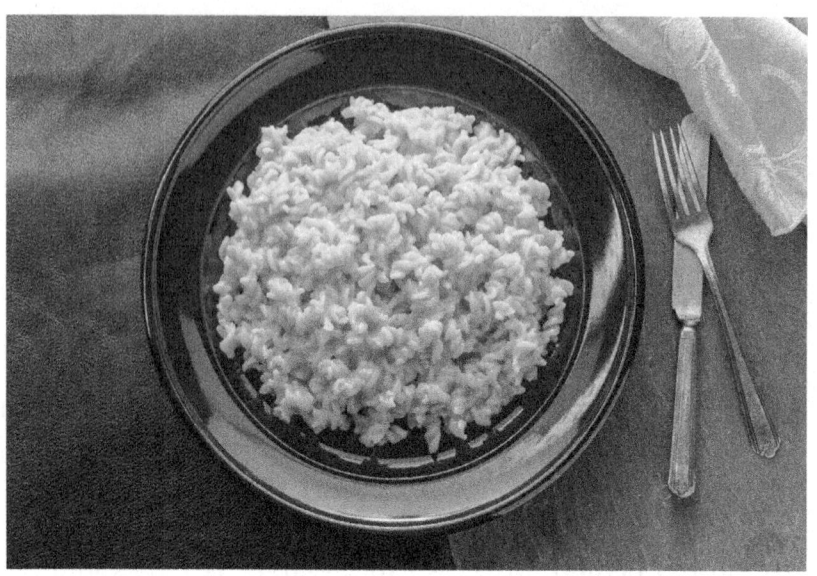

Cooking Time: 50 Minutes + 8-12 Hours for soaking

Serving Size: 8-10 Servings

Ingredients

- 12 ounces of any alkaline pasta
- 1/4 cup of Chickpea Flour
- 1 cup of raw Brazil Nuts
- 1/2 teaspoon of Ground Achiote
- 2 teaspoons of Onion Powder
- 1 teaspoon of Pure Sea Salt
- 2 teaspoons of Grape Seed Oil

- 1 cup of *Homemade Hempseed Milk (see recipe on page 132)**
- 1 cup of Spring Water + extra for soaking
- juice from 1/2 Key Lime

Cooking Instructions

1. Put Brazil Nuts in a medium bowl and cover them with Spring Water. Soak overnight.
2. Cook your favorite alkaline pasta.
3. Preheat your oven to 350 degrees Fahrenheit.
4. Place the cooked pasta in a baking dish and drizzle extra Grape Seed Oil to prevent it sticking to the bottom.
5. Add all ingredients to a blender and blend for 2 to 4 minutes until smooth.
6. Pour the brazil nut sauce over the macaroni and mix well.
7. Put the baking dish in the oven and bake for about 30 minutes. **
8. Serve and enjoy your Macaroni and Cheese!

Useful Tips

* If you don't have prepared *Homemade Hempseed Milk*, add Coconut Milk instead.

** If you want to make the top crispy, broil the pasta for about 5 minutes.

Healthy Fried-Rice

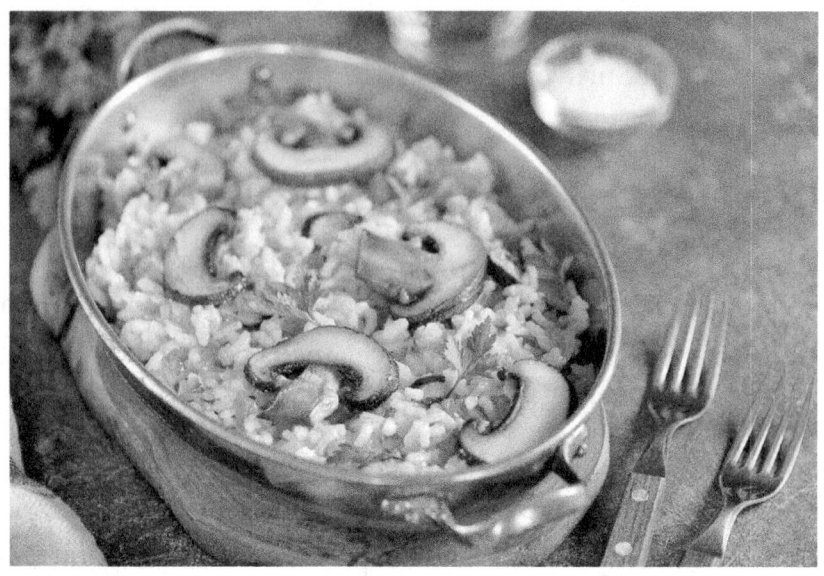

Cooking Time: 20 Minutes + 30 Minutes (for boiling)

Serving Size: 2 Servings

Ingredients

- 1 cup of cooked Wild Rice*
- 1/2 cup of sliced Mushrooms
- 1/2 cup of cubed Zucchini
- 1/2 cup of cubed Bell Peppers
- 1/4 diced Onion
- Pure Sea Salt, to taste
- Cayenne Powder, to taste
- 1/2 tablespoon of Grape Seed Oil

Cooking Instructions

1. Heat Grape Seed Oil in a medium pan over medium heat.
2. Add diced Onion to the pan and sauté until golden brown.
3. Add the Mushrooms, Zucchini and Bell Peppers and cook for 5 more minutes. The vegetables should become a little softer.
4. Add boiled Wild Rice to the pan and continue sautéing until lightly browned.
5. Serve and enjoy your Healthy Fried-Rice!

Useful Tips

* If you want, you can use cooked Quinoa instead.

Meatballs

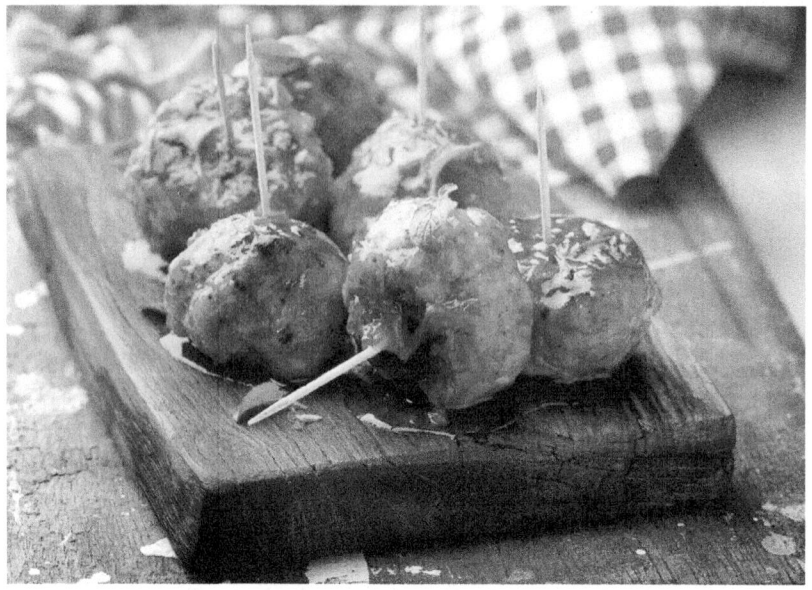

Cooking Time: 30 Minutes

Serving Size: 7-9 Servings

Ingredients

- 1 1/2 cups of cooked Garbanzo Beans
- 1 cup of Garbanzo Bean Flour
- 2 cups of Mushrooms
- 1/4 cup of diced Green Peppers
- 1/2 cup of diced Onions
- 2 teaspoons of Oregano
- 1 tablespoon of Onion Powder
- 2 teaspoons of Basil
- 1 teaspoon of Fennel Powder
- 1 teaspoon of Dill

- 1 teaspoon of Savory
- 1 teaspoon of Sage
- 1/2 teaspoon of Ginger Powder
- 1/2 teaspoon of Ground Cloves
- 1 teaspoon of Pure Sea Salt
- 1/2 teaspoon of Cayenne Powder
- 6 cups of *Fragrant Tomato Sauce (see recipe on page 118)*
- 2 tablespoons of Grape Seed Oil

Cooking Instructions

1. Place Mushrooms, cooked Garbanzo Beans, Onions, Green Peppers and seasonings into a food processor. Blend them well for 1 minute.
2. Add blended mixture to a large bowl and mix in Garbanzo Bean Flour. Try to make balls. If balls do not form, add more flour.
3. Shape the meatballs and let them rest for a couple minutes.
4. Add Grape Seed Oil to a skillet and warm it on medium heat.
5. Place a couple of meatballs on the skillet. Cook for 2 minutes on each side.
6. Add *Fragrant Tomato Sauce* to the meatballs and simmer for additional 5 minutes.
7. Serve* and enjoy your Meatballs!

Useful Tips

*You can serve it with our *Flatbread (see recipe on page 146)* or *Homemade Pasta (see recipe on page 100)*.

Zucchini Noodles with Avocado Sauce

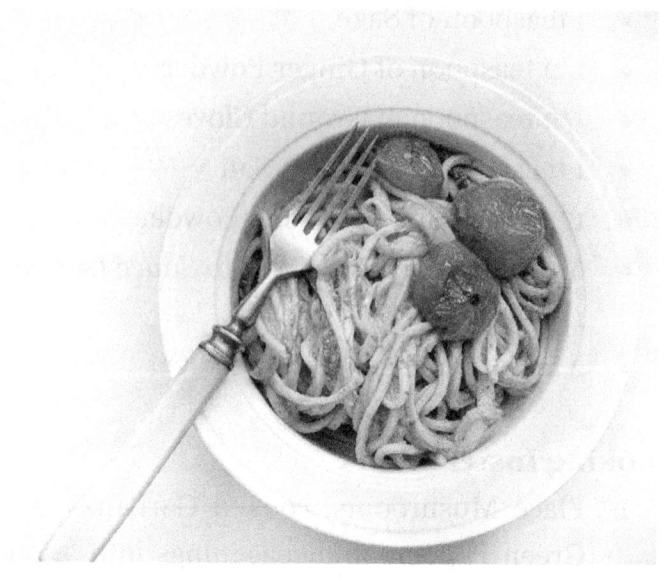

Cooking Time: 30 Minutes

Serving Size: 3 Servings

Ingredients

- 3 Medium Zucchini
- 1 1/2 cup of Cherry Tomatoes
- 1 Avocado
- 2 sliced Green Onions
- 1/3 cup of fresh leaf Parsley
- 3 tablespoons of Olive Oil
- juice of 1 Key Lime
- 1 tablespoon of Spring Water

- Pure Sea Salt, to taste
- Cayenne, to taste

Cooking Instructions

1. Preheat your oven to 400 degrees Fahrenheit.
2. Cover a baking sheet with a piece of parchment paper.
3. Put the Cherry Tomatoes on the covered baking sheet. Drizzle with 1 tablespoon of Olive Oil and season with Pure Sea Salt and Cayenne.
4. Bake the Tomatoes for about 15 to 20 minutes until they start to split.
5. Add quartered Avocado, torn Parsley leaves, sliced Green Onions, Spring Water, Key Lime Juice and 1/2 teaspoon of Pure Sea Salt to a food processor. Blend until it achieves a creamy consistency. If the sauce is too thick, add more Spring Water.
6. Cut off the ends of the Zucchini. Using a spiralizer, make zucchini noodles.
7. Mix the zucchini noodles with the prepared avocado sauce.
8. Divide into 3 small bowls and serve with Cherry Tomatoes.
9. Enjoy your Zucchini Noodles with Avocado Sauce!

Vegetarian Fajitas

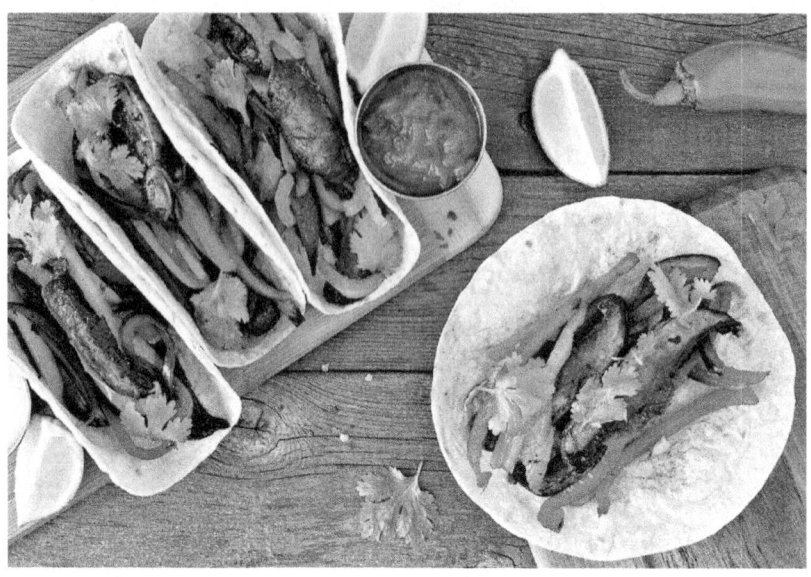

Cooking Time: 20 Minutes

Serving Size: 3 Servings

Ingredients

- 6 *Tortillas (see recipe on page 150)*
- 3 Large Portobello Mushrooms
- 1 Onion
- 2 Bell Peppers
- 1 teaspoon of Onion Powder
- 1 teaspoon of Habanero
- 1/8 teaspoon of Cayenne Powder

- juice of 1/2 Key Lime
- 1 tablespoon of Grape Seed Oil

Cooking Instructions

1. Rinse the Portobello Mushrooms and remove their stems. Cut into 1/3-inch slices.
2. Cut Onion and Bell Peppers into thin slices.
3. Add Grape Seed Oil to a large skillet and warm on medium heat. Add sliced Onions and Bell Peppers and cook for 2 minutes.
4. Place sliced Mushrooms and seasonings into the pan. Cook for 7 to 8 minutes, stirring occasionally. Remove from the heat.
5. Grab a small pan, put *Tortillas* on it and warm for 30 to 60 seconds on each side.
6. Place the filling mixture into the *Tortillas'* center and sprinkle the Key Lime juice over the vegetables.
7. Serve* and enjoy your Vegetarian Fajitas!

Useful Tips

* You can serve it with our *Fragrant Tomato Sauce (see recipe on page 118)* or *Avocado Sauce (see recipe on page 116)*.

Homemade Hummus

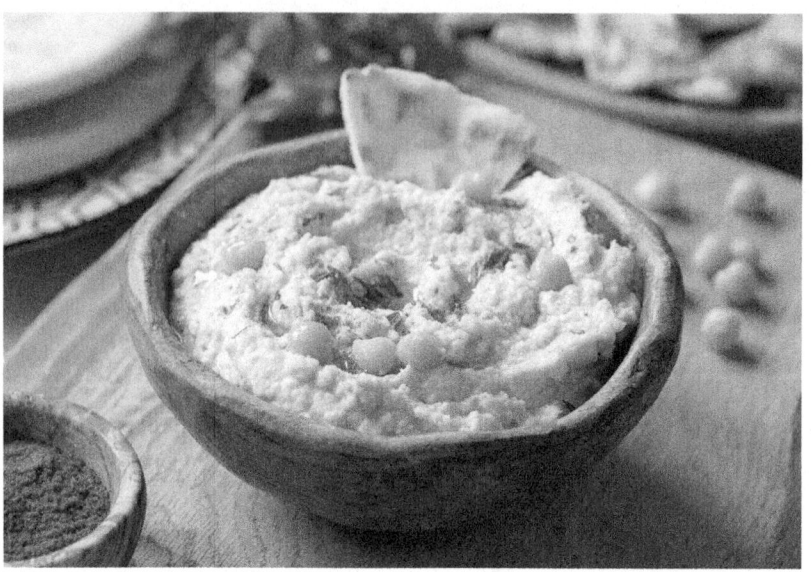

Cooking Time: 10 Minutes

Serving Size: 1 to 2 cups

Ingredients

- 1/3 cup of Raw Sesame "Tahini" Butter
- 1 cup of cooked Garbanzo Beans
- 1/2 teaspoon of Onion Powder
- Pure Sea Salt, to taste
- 2 tablespoons of Olive Oil
- 2 tablespoons of Key Lime Juice

Cooking Instructions

1. Take a food processor.*
2. Blend all the ingredients thoroughly until it reaches a creamy consistency.
3. Serve and enjoy your Homemade Hummus!

Useful Tips

* If you don't have the food processor, you can blend with a high-powered blender.

** You can serve it with our *Flatbread (see recipe on page 146), Tortillas (see recipe on page 150), Tortilla Chips (see recipe on page 152),* or *Healthy Crackers (see recipe on page 148).*

Zucchini Hummus Wrap

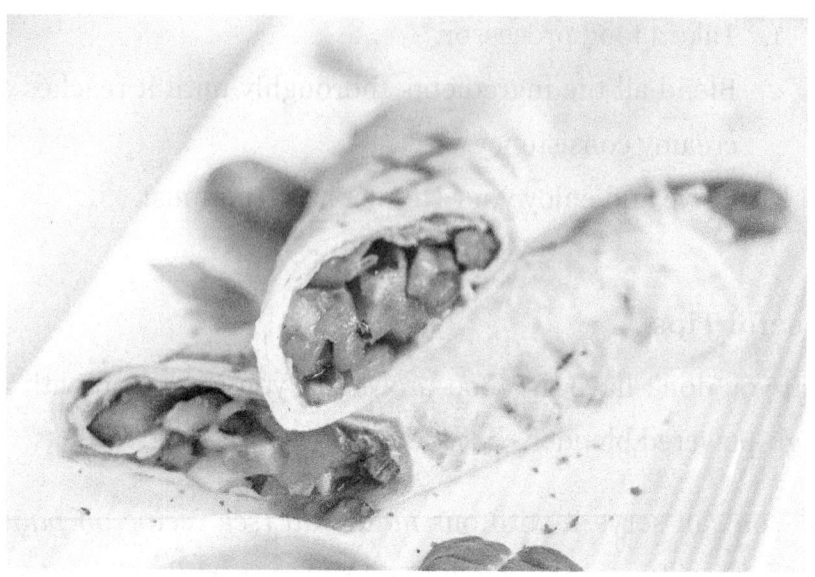

Cooking Time: 15 Minutes

Serving Size: 2 Servings

Ingredients

- 2 *Tortillas (see recipe on page 150)*
- 4 tablespoons of *Homemade Hummus (see recipe on page 82)*
- 1 sliced Zucchini
- 1 cup of Romaine Lettuce*
- 1 sliced Plum Tomato**
- 1/4 sliced Red Onion
- Pure Sea Salt, to taste
- Cayenne, to taste

The Doctor Sebi Diet: The Complete Guide to a Plant-Based Diet

- 1 tablespoon of Grape Seed Oil

Cooking Instructions

1. Warm a grill pan*** with Grape Seed Oil on medium heat.
2. Add sliced Zucchini to the pan and season with Pure Sea Salt and Cayenne.
3. Cook on medium heat for about 3 minutes then flip and cook for an additional 2 minutes. Remove it from the heat.
4. Put the *Tortillas* on the grill for 1 minute each until they warm. Remove them from the grill.
5. Make wraps. Take a warm *Tortilla* and place in the center 2 tablespoons of *Homemade Hummus*, 1/2 cup of greens, Onion, Tomato and Zucchini slices.
6. Wrap it tightly and serve.****
7. Enjoy your Zucchini Hummus Wrap!

Useful Tips

* If you don't want to use Romaine Lettuce, add Wild Arugula instead.

** If you don't have Plum Tomatoes, you can add 6 Cherry Tomatoes instead.

*** If you don't have a grill, cook on a skillet pan.

**** You can serve it with our *"Cheese" Sauce (see recipe on page 120), Sweet Barbecue Sauce (see recipe on page 114),* or *Fragrant Tomato Sauce (see recipe on page 118).*

Sausage Links

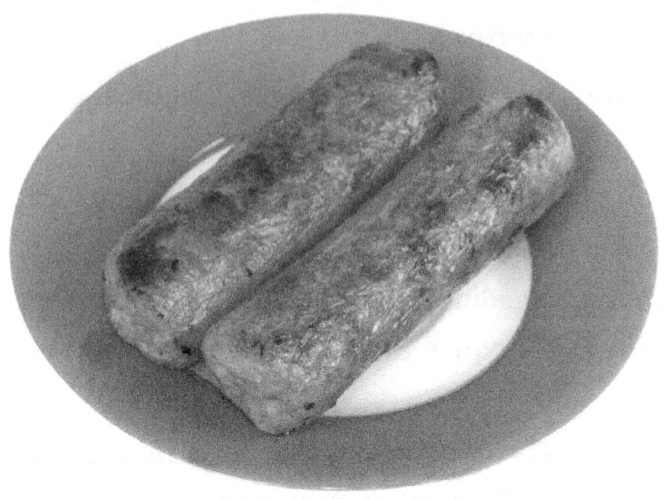

Cooking Time: 30 Minutes

Serving Size: 8-10 Servings

Ingredients
- 2 cups of cooked Garbanzo Beans
- 1 quartered Roma Tomato
- 1 cup quartered Mushrooms
- 1/2 cup of chopped Onion
- 1/2 cup of Garbanzo Bean Flour
- 1 tablespoon of Onion Powder
- 1 teaspoon of Ground Sage
- 1 teaspoon of Basil
- 1 teaspoon of Oregano

- 1 teaspoon of Dill
- ½ teaspoon Ground Cloves
- 1 teaspoon of Pure Sea Salt
- ½ teaspoon of Cayenne Powder
- 2 tablespoons of Grape Seed Oil

Cooking Instructions

1. Put all the ingredients, except the Garbanzo Bean Flour and grape seed oil, into a food processor.
2. Blend for 15 seconds.
3. Add the Garbanzo Bean Flour to the mixture and blend for 30 more seconds until well combined.
4. Put the mixture into a piping bag and cut a small piece from the bottom corner.
5. Add Grape Seed Oil to a skillet and warm on high heat.
6. Reduce to medium heat. Squeeze out the prepared mixture into the pan to form sausages.
7. Cook them for about 3 to 4 minutes on all sides. Turn carefully to prevent them falling apart.
8. Serve* and enjoy your Sausage Links!

Useful Tips

* You can serve it with our *"Cheese" Sauce (see recipe on page 120), Sweet Barbecue Sauce (see recipe on page 114),* or *Fragrant Tomato Sauce (see recipe on page 118)*.

Garbanzo Bean Burger

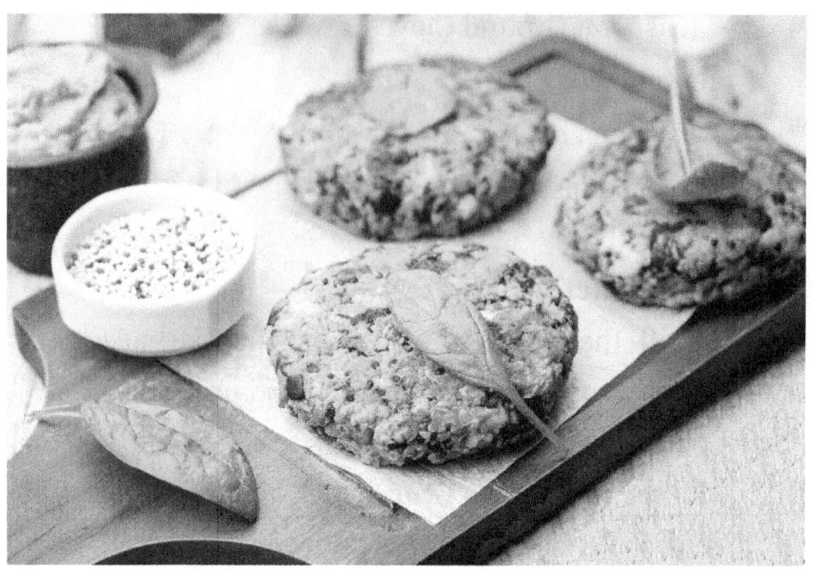

Cooking Time: 40 Minutes

Serving Size: 3-4 Servings

Ingredients

Cutlet:

- 1 cup of Garbanzo Bean Flour
- 1 diced Plum Tomato
- 1/2 cup of diced Kale
- 1/2 cup of diced Green Peppers
- 1/2 cup of minced Onions
- 2 teaspoons od Onion Powder

- 2 teaspoons of Oregano
- 2 teaspoons of Basil
- 1 teaspoon of Dill
- 1/2 teaspoon of Cayenne
- 2 teaspoons of Pure Sea Salt
- 1/2 teaspoon of Cayenne Powder
- 2 tablespoons of Grape Seed Oil
- 1/4 to 1/2 cup of Spring Water

Burger:

- 8 *Flatbreads (see recipe on page 146)*
- 2 sliced Plum Tomatoes
- 1 sliced Red Onion
- 1 cup of sauce*

Cooking Instructions

1. Mix all vegetables and seasonings in a large bowl.
2. Add the Garbanzo Bean Flour to it and mix well.
3. Slowly pour Spring Water and mix thoroughly until it can be easily shaped into cutlets. If it's too loose, add more flour.
4. Add Grape Seed Oil to a skillet and warm it on high heat.

5. Reduce to medium heat. Place the formed cutlets in the pan and cook for about 2 to 3 minutes on all sides until golden brown.
6. Take one *Flatbread* and put the cooked burger cutlet on it. Add greens, sliced Tomatoes, Onions and any sauce from our recipes.*
7. Serve and enjoy your Garbanzo Bean Burger!

Useful Tips

* You can serve it with our *"Cheese" Sauce (see recipe on page 120), Sweet Barbecue Sauce (see recipe on page 114), Fragrant Tomato Sauce (see recipe on page 118),* or *Avocado Sauce (see recipe on page 116).*

Margherita Pizza

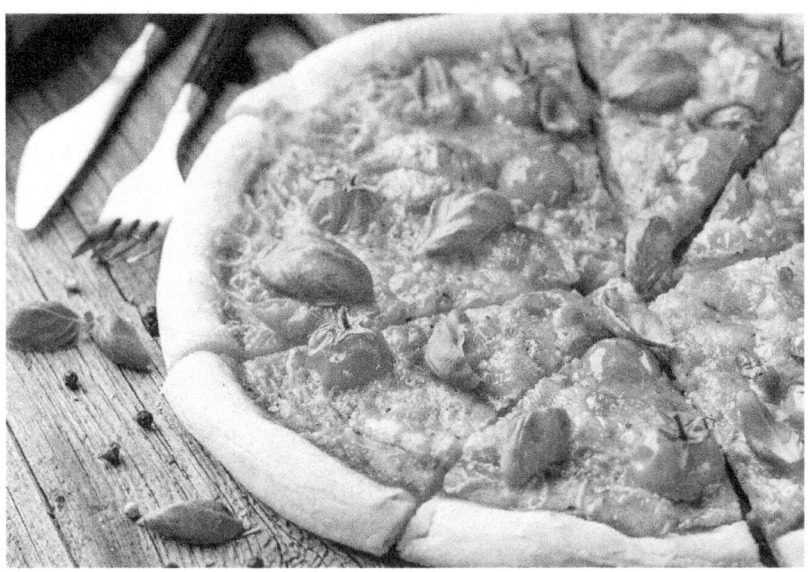

Cooking Time: 1 Hour

Serving Size: 4 Servings

Ingredients

Crust:

- 1 1/2 cups of Spelt Flour
- 1/2 teaspoon of Pure Sea Salt
- 1/2 teaspoon of Basil
- 1/2 teaspoon of Oregano
- 1/2 teaspoon of Onion Powder
- 1 cup of Spring Water

Cheese:

- 1 cup of soaked Brazil Nuts (overnight or for at least 3 hours)
- 1 teaspoon of Sea Moss Gel *(check information on page 18)*
- 1/2 teaspoon of Basil
- 1/2 teaspoon of Oregano
- 1/2 teaspoon of Onion Powder
- 1/4 teaspoon of Pure Sea Salt
- 1/4 cup of *Homemade Hempseed Milk (see recipe on page 132)**
- 1 teaspoon of Key Lime Juice
- 1/2 cup of Spring Water

Toppings:

- Sliced Plum or Cherry Tomatoes
- Chopped Fresh Basil
- Sliced Red Onions
- *"Garlic" Sauce (see recipe on page 124)*

Cooking Instructions

1. Preheat your oven to 350 degrees Fahrenheit.
2. In a medium bowl, add Spelt Flour and seasonings and mix well. Pour 1/2 cup of Spring Water and mix.

Continue adding more water until dough can be formed into a ball.

3. Prepare your working space and spread flour on the surface. Roll the dough out with a rolling pin, adding more flour as necessary to avoid sticking.
4. Spread the dough out on a baking sheet, brush with Grape Seed Oil, and make holes with a fork. Place in the oven and bake 10 to 15 minutes.
5. Add all ingredients for the cheese to a blender. Blend well until consistency is smooth.
6. Take the dough out from the oven. Spread with *"Garlic" Sauce* and prepared cheese. Top the pizza with sliced Tomatoes, Onions, Basil, and more cheese on the top.
7. Bake on the bottom rack for 10 to 15 minutes at 425 degrees Fahrenheit.
8. Serve and enjoy your Margherita Pizza!

Useful Tips

*If you don't have *Homemade Hempseed Milk*, you can substitute *Homemade Walnut Milk (see recipe on page 128)*.

Ravioli

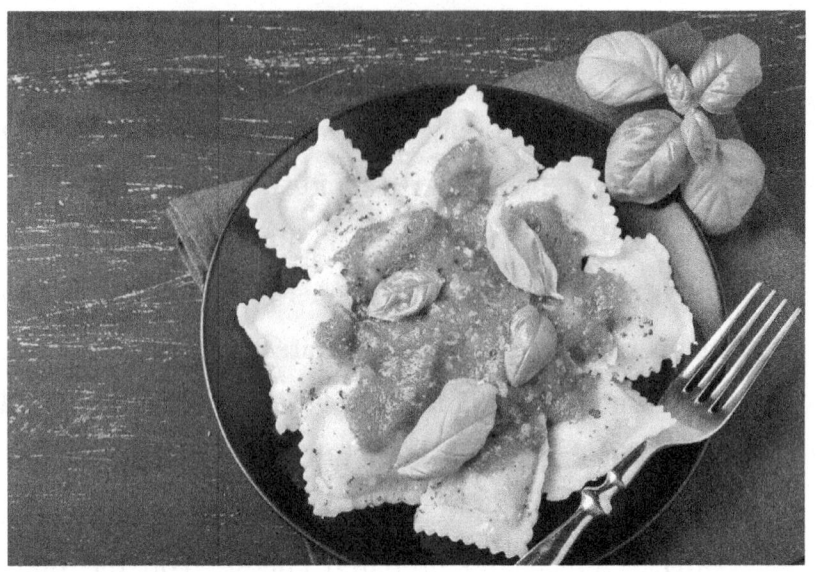

Cooking Time: 1 Hour

Serving Size: 5 Servings

Ingredients

Filling:

- 1 cup of Chickpea Flour
- 1 quartered Roma Tomato
- 2 cups of quartered Mushrooms
- 1 cup of chopped Kale
- 1/3 cup of diced Onions
- 1 cup of diced Green and Red Bell Peppers

- 1 tablespoon of Onion Powder
- 1 teaspoon of Ginger
- 2 teaspoons of Oregano
- 2 teaspoons of Dill
- 2 teaspoons of Basil
- 2 teaspoons of Thyme
- 1 teaspoon of Pure Sea Salt
- 1/2 teaspoon of Cayenne

Dough:
- 1/2 cup of Chickpea Flour
- 1 1/2 cups of Spelt Flour
- 1/2 teaspoon of Oregano
- 1/2 teaspoon of Basil
- 1 teaspoon of Pure Sea Salt
- 3/4 cup of Spring Water

Cheese:
- 1/2 cup of soaked Brazil Nuts (overnight or for at least 3 hours)
- 2 teaspoons of Onion Powder
- 1/2 teaspoon of Oregano
- 1 teaspoon of Pure Sea Salt
- 1/2 teaspoon of Cayenne Powder
- 1/2 cup of Spring Water

Cooking Instructions

1. Blend all filling ingredients, except the Chickpea Flour, in a food processor for 30 to 40 seconds.
2. Add Chickpea Flour to the mixture and blend until well combined.
3. Add Grape Seed Oil to a skillet and warm on high heat.
4. Reduce to medium heat. Spread out the ravioli filling to the skillet and cook for 3 to 4 minutes on all sides.
5. Break up the filling and cook for 3 more minutes, then transfer it to a medium bowl.
6. Add all ingredients for the cheese to the food processor and blend until consistency is creamy. If it's too thick, add some Spring Water.
7. Mix the filling with the cheese mixture in the bowl.
8. Put all the dry ingredients for the dough in the food processor and blend for 10 to 20 seconds. Slowly add Spring Water while blending until dough can be shaped into a ball.
9. Spread flour on the working space. Take 1/4 of the dough and roll it out into a thin sheet.
10. Place rounded teaspoonfuls of filling and cheese 1 inch apart on one side of the dough. Fold the dough over and press together around the filling to seal. Cut it into individual ravioli with a pastry cutter or knife.

11. Repeat steps 9 and 10 with the remaining dough and filling.
12. Bring a pot of Spring Water to a boil. Add a little Pure Sea Salt and Grape Seed Oil, then cook the ravioli for about 4 to 6 minutes.
13. Strain and serve*.
14. Enjoy your Ravioli!

Useful Tips

* You can serve it with *Fragrant Tomato Sauce (see recipe on page 118)*.

Chickpea French Fries

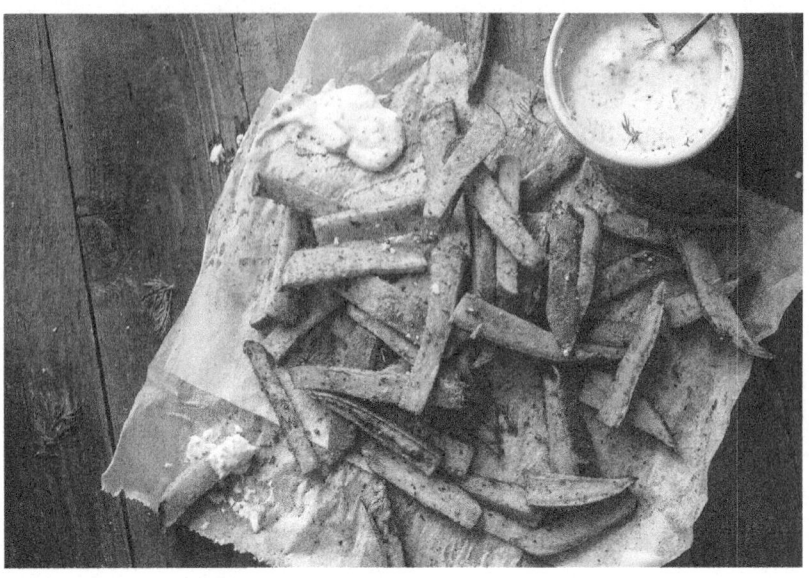

Cooking Time: 1 Hour 40 Minutes

Serving Size: 4-8 Servings

Ingredients
- 2 cups of Chickpea Flour
- 1/2 cup of diced Green Bell Peppers
- 1/2 cup of minced Onions
- 1 tablespoon of Oregano
- 1 tablespoon of Onion Powder
- 1 tablespoon of Pure Sea Salt
- 1 teaspoon of Cayenne
- 4 cups of Spring Water
- 2 tablespoons of Grape Seed Oil

Cooking Instructions

1. Boil the Spring Water in a large pot.
2. Reduce to medium heat and whisk in Chickpea Flour.
3. Add minced Onions, diced Green Bell Peppers, and seasonings to the pot. Cook for 10 minutes, stirring occasionally, until it thickens.
4. Cover a baking sheet with a piece of parchment paper and grease with a little Grape Seed Oil.
5. Pour the batter on the sheet, spread with a spatula, and cover with another lightly greased piece of parchment paper.
6. Put the baking sheet in the freezer for about 20 minutes.
7. Remove from the freezer and cut the batter into fry shaped pieces.
8. Preheat your oven to 400 degrees Fahrenheit.
9. Cover a baking sheet with a piece of parchment paper and lightly grease.
10. Put the French fries on the baking sheet.
11. Bake for about 20 minutes then flip them over and continue baking for 15 more minutes until golden brown.
12. Serve* and enjoy your Chickpea French Fries!

Useful Tips

* You can serve it with *"Cheese" Sauce (see recipe on page 120)* or *Fragrant Tomato Sauce (see recipe on page 118)*.

Homemade Pasta

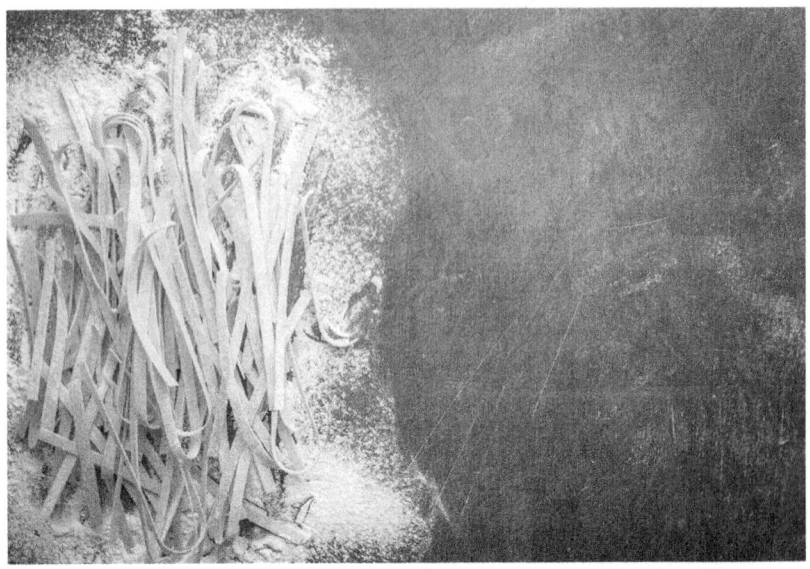

Cooking Time: 50 Minutes

Serving Size: 4 Servings

Ingredients
- 2 cups of Spelt Flour
- 1/2 teaspoon of Pure Sea Salt
- 3/4 cup of warm Spring Water
- 2 tablespoons of Grape Seed Oil

Cooking Instructions
1. In a large bowl, mix together 3/4 cup of warm Spring Water, 1 cup of Spelt Flour and Pure Sea Salt until it can be shaped into a ball.

2. Spread flour on your work space.
3. Knead the dough for 5 to 8 minutes.
4. Make a ball and cover it first with flour then plastic wrap. Set aside for 15-20 minutes.
5. Unwrap the dough and divide into 4 equal parts.
6. Take 1 part you are going to work with. Re-wrap the 3 other parts.
7. Roll the dough out in one direction a couple of times with a rolling pin, then flip it and repeat the rolling process. Remember to add more flour when flipping.
8. Cut the dough into individual pieces of pasta using a pastry cutter.
9. Repeat steps 6, 7, and 8 with the remaining dough.
10. Pour Spring Water and Pure Sea Salt into a large pot and bring to a boil.
11. Cook pasta in the boiling water for 1 to 2 minutes then strain.
12. Serve** and enjoy your Homemade Pasta!

Useful Tips

* If you don't have Spelt Flour, you can add Kamut Flour instead.

** You can serve it with our *"Cheese" Sauce (see recipe on page 120), Sweet Barbecue Sauce (see recipe on page 114),* or *Fragrant Tomato Sauce (see recipe on page 118).*

Vegetarian Lasagna

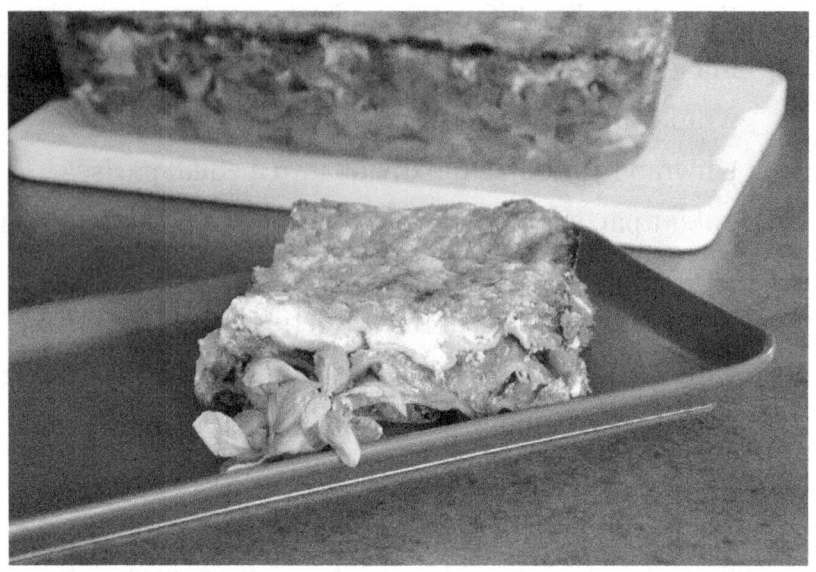

Cooking Time: 3 Hours 20 Minutes

Serving Size: 6-8 Servings

Ingredients

Pasta:

- Lasagna Sheets from Spelt Flour*

Tomato Sauce:

- 12 quartered Plum Tomatoes
- 1 tablespoon of Onion Powder
- 2 teaspoons of Oregano
- 2 teaspoons of Basil

- 1 tablespoon of Agave Syrup
- 2 teaspoons of Pure Sea Salt
- 1/2 teaspoon of Cayenne

"Meat":
- 1 cup of cooked Garbanzo Beans
- 2 cups of cooked Spelt Berries
- 1/2 cup of *"Garlic" Sauce (see recipe on page 124)*
- 1 cup of diced Red, Yellow and Green Bell Peppers
- 1 cup of minced Onions
- 1 teaspoon of Fennel Powder
- 2 tablespoons of Onion Powder
- 2 teaspoons of Basil
- 2 teaspoons of Oregano
- 1 tablespoon of Pure Sea Salt

Cheese:
- 2 cups of soaked Brazil Nuts (overnight or for at least 3 hours)
- 1 tablespoon of Hemp Seeds
- 1 teaspoon of Oregano
- 1 tablespoon of Onion Powder
- 1 teaspoon of Basil
- 1 teaspoon of Pure Sea Salt
- 1 cup of Spring Water

Extras:

- Sliced Zucchini
- Sliced Mushrooms
- Grape Seed Oil

Cooking Instructions

1. Preheat your oven to 350 degrees Fahrenheit.
2. Put all ingredients for the tomato sauce in a blender. Blend for 2 to 3 minutes until well combined.
3. Pour it into a saucepan and first bring to a boil then reduce to low heat. Simmer, stirring occasionally, for 2 hours until thickened.
4. To prepare the "meat" mixture, blend cooked Garbanzo Beans, seasonings, and cooked Spelt Berries in your food processor until smooth.
5. Add Grape Seed Oil to a skillet and warm on high heat.
6. Add diced Bell Peppers and minced Onions and sauté for about 5 minutes.
7. Add Garbanzo Bean/Spelt mixture and *"Garlic" Sauce* to the skillet pan and continue cooking for 10 to 12 minutes until golden brown.
8. Add all ingredients for the cheese to a blender. Blend well until consistency is smooth. Add 1/4 cup of Spring Water if it is too thick.

9. Reserve 1 cup of tomato sauce. Add the remaining sauce to the "meat" mixture and mix well.
10. Slice Zucchini and Mushrooms lengthwise.
11. Take a 9x13 glass baking dish and spread some tomato sauce on the bottom to prevent sticking.
12. Layer the dish in the following order: Lasagna Sheets, sliced Mushrooms and Zucchini, cheese and "meat" mixture, then Lasagna Sheets once again.
13. Repeat the last step until you have 4 layers of pasta.
14. Cover the last layer with the "meat" mixture and cheese. Pour some tomato sauce over the top.
15. Bake in the oven for about 35 to 45 minutes until cooked.
16. Serve and enjoy your Vegetarian Lasagna!

Useful Tips

*If you don't have Spelt Lasagna Sheets, you can make some yourself using our recipe *Homemade Pasta (see recipe on page 100)*.

Kamut Cereal

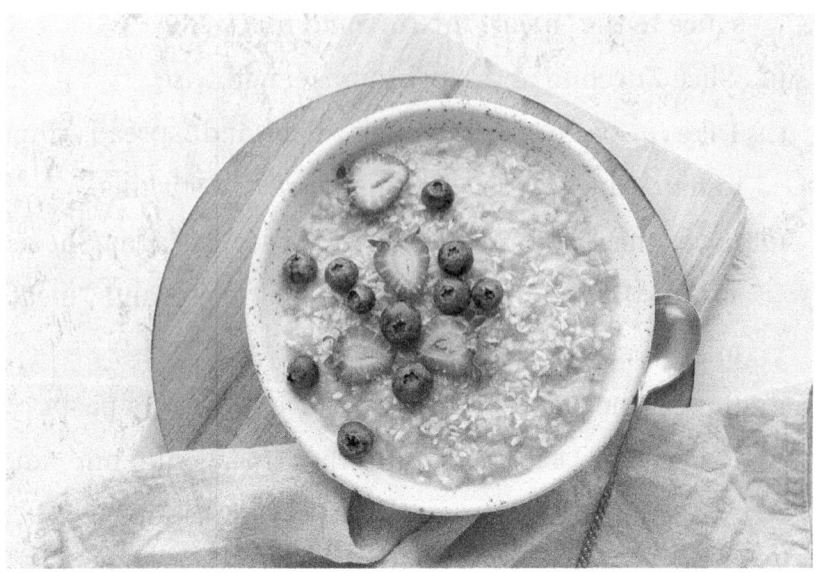

Cooking Time: 15 Minutes

Serving Size: 2 Servings

Ingredients

- 1 cup of Kamut
- Oregano, to taste
- Onion Powder, to taste (optional)
- Pure Sea Salt, to taste (optional)
- Cayenne, to taste (optional)
- Fruits*
- 2 cups of Spring Water

Cooking Instructions

1. Add 2 cups of Spring Water and a pinch of Pure Sea Salt to a saucepan and bring to a boil.
2. Add Kamut Berries to a food processor. Grind until it resembles flour.
3. Add the grinded Kamut to the saucepan and stir from time to time.
4. If it is too thick, add more Spring Water to achieve the desired consistency.
5. Add seasonings or any fruits* you desire.
6. Serve and enjoy your Kamut Cereal!

Useful Tips

* You can add any fruits from Doctor Sebi's Food List.

Vegan "Ribs"

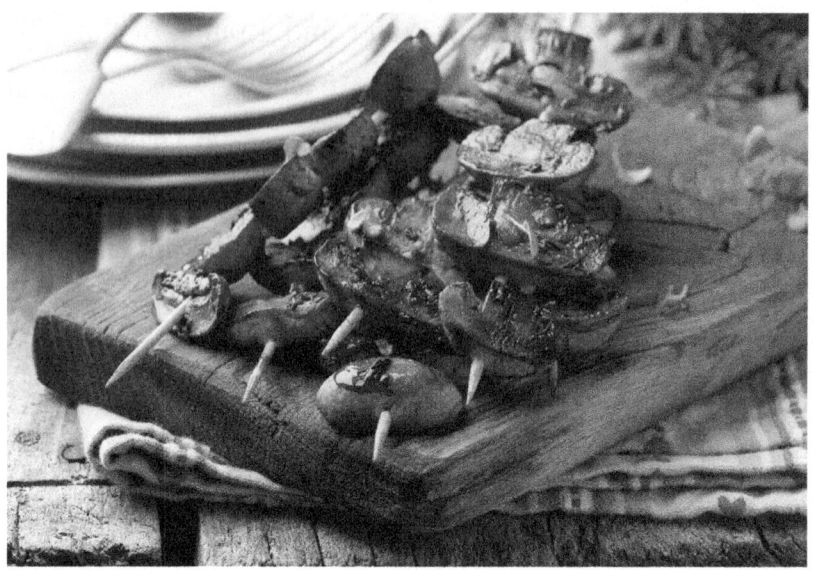

Cooking Time: 50 Minutes

Serving Size: 1 Person

Ingredients

- 2 Portobello Mushrooms
- 1/2 cup of *Sweet Barbecue Sauce (see recipe on page 114)*
- 1 teaspoon of Onion Powder
- 1 teaspoon of Pure Sea Salt
- 1/2 teaspoon of Cayenne Powder
- 1/4 cup of Spring Water
- 2 tablespoons of Grape Seed Oil

Cooking Instructions

1. Remove the gills from the Portobello Mushrooms and cut them into 1/2-inch thick slices.
2. Put the sliced Mushrooms, Spring Water, *Sweet Barbecue Sauce*, and seasonings into a large container with a sealable lid.
3. Shake the container and leave it in a refrigerator for about 6 to 7 hours. Flip the container over every 2 hours.
4. Take 3 to 4 Mushroom slices and thread a skewer through their centers.
5. Repeat until all the slices are on skewers.
6. Add Grape Seed Oil to a griddle or skillet and warm on medium heat.
7. Cook mushroom ribs for 13 to 15 minutes, flipping them every 3 minutes.
8. Serve and enjoy your Vegan "Ribs"!

Stuffed Bell Peppers

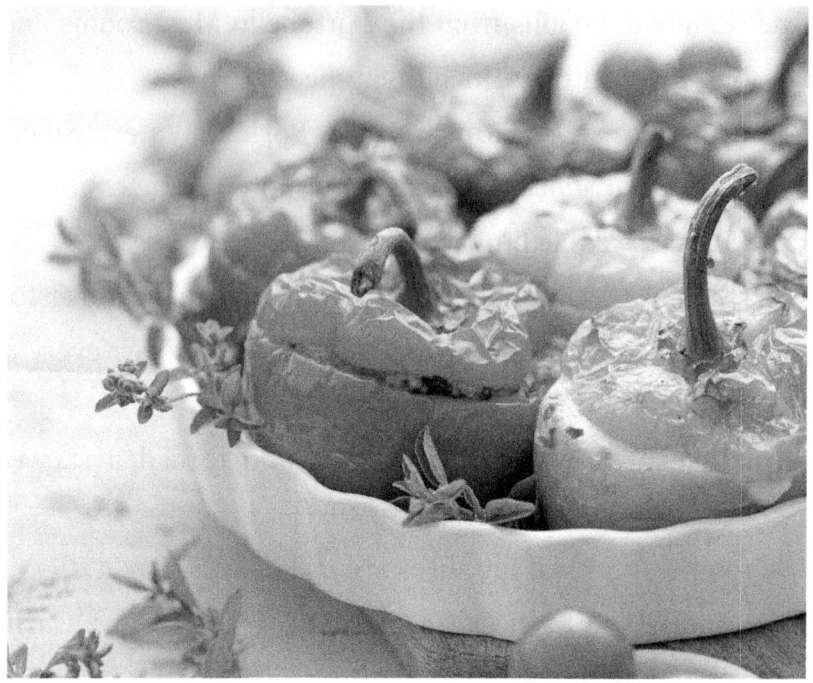

Cooking Time: 1 Hour

Serving Size: 4-6 Servings

Ingredients
- 4 to 6 Bell Peppers
- 2 diced Plum Tomatoes
- 1 cup of sliced Mushrooms
- 1/2 minced Red Onion
- 1/2 minced White Onion
- 2 cups of cooked Wild Rice

- 1 teaspoon of Onion Powder
- 1 teaspoon of Oregano
- 1 teaspoon of Pure Sea Salt
- 1/2 teaspoon of Cayenne
- 2 tablespoons of Grape Seed Oil
- 1 cup of *Fragrant Tomato Sauce (see recipe on page 118)*
- 1 1/2 cups of *"Cheese" Sauce (see recipe on page 120)*
- Spring Water

Cooking Instructions

1. Preheat your oven to 350 degrees Fahrenheit.

Peppers:

2. Cut off the top of the Bell Peppers, remove the seeds and flesh.
3. Place Peppers in a medium bowl and cover them with hot or boiling Spring Water. Wait for about 5 minutes until they are soft.
4. Remove from the water and place upright in a baking dish. Sprinkle 1 teaspoon of Pure Sea Salt on them.

Filling:

5. Add Grape Seed Oil to a skillet and warm on high heat.

6. Reduce to medium heat. Add sliced Mushrooms, minced Onions, and seasonings then mix.
7. Sauté for about 5 minutes.
8. Add cooked Wild Rice, diced Plum Tomatoes, 1/2 cup of *Fragrant Tomato Sauce,* and 1 cup of *"Cheese" Sauce* to the vegetables and mix well.
9. Simmer for 5 minutes.

10. Stuff prepared Peppers with the filling mixture and spread the remaining sauces on top.
11. Bake the stuffed peppers in the oven for 25 to 30 minutes until cooked.
12. Serve and enjoy your Stuffed Bell Peppers!

SAUCES

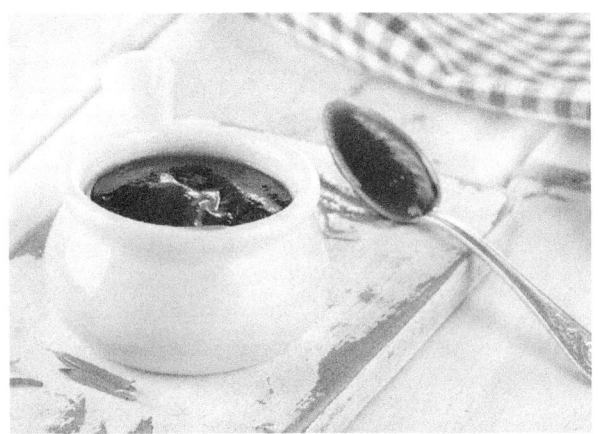

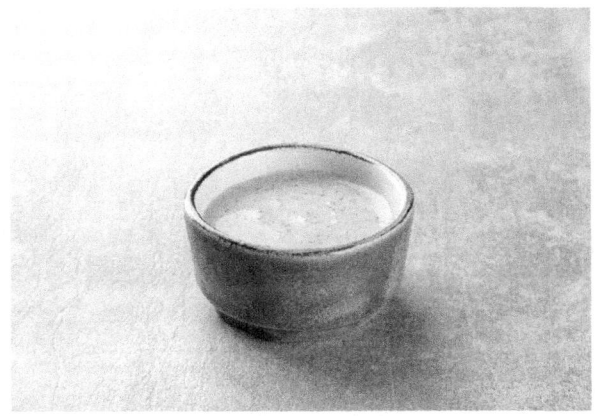

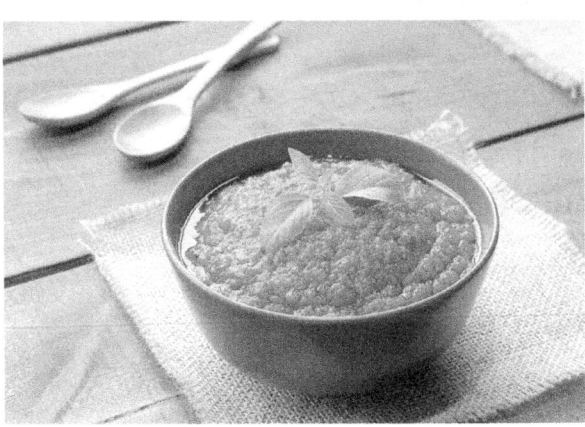

Sweet Barbecue Sauce

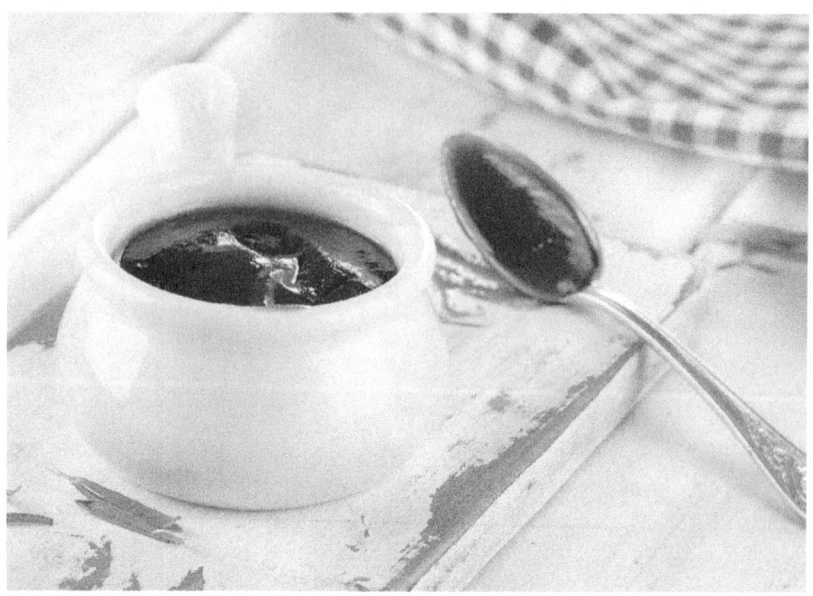

Cooking Time: 40 Minutes

Serving Size: 1 Cup

Ingredients

- 6 quartered Plum Tomatoes
- 1/4 cup of chopped White Onions
- 1/4 cup of Date Sugar
- 2 teaspoons f Pure Sea Salt
- 2 tablespoons of Agave Syrup
- 1/4 teaspoon of Cayenne
- 2 teaspoons of Onion Powder

- 1/2 teaspoon of Ground Ginger
- 1/8 teaspoon of Cloves

Cooking Instructions

1. Add all ingredients, excluding Date Sugar, to a blender and blend them thoroughly.
2. Pour mixture into a saucepan and add Date Sugar.
3. Cook over medium heat, stirring occasionally to prevent sticking until boiling.
4. Reduce heat to a simmer. Cover the saucepan with a lid and cook for 15 minutes, stirring from time to time.
5. Use an immersion blender to blend the sauce until it is smooth.
6. Continue to cook at low heat until sauce thickens (about 10 minutes).
7. Allow mixture to cool before using.
8. Serve and enjoy your Sweet Barbecue Sauce!

Avocado Sauce

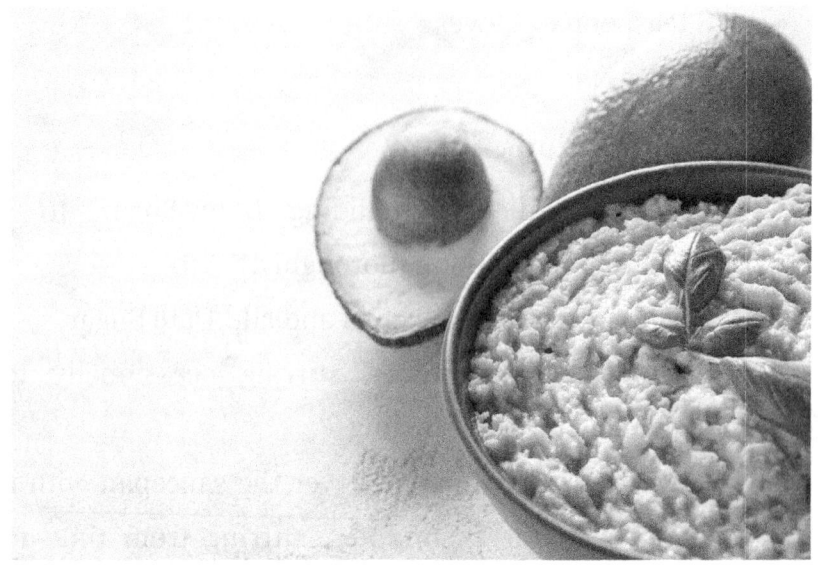

Cooking Time: 10 Minutes

Serving Size: 1 Cup

Ingredients

- 1 ripe Avocado
- 1 pinch of Basil
- 1/2 teaspoon of Oregano
- 1/2 teaspoon of Onion Powder
- 2 tablespoons of minced Onion
- 1/2 teaspoon of Pure Sea Walt

Cooking Instructions

1. Cut the Avocado in half, peel it, and remove the seed.
2. Chop it into small pieces and throw into a food processor.
3. Add all other ingredients and blend for 2 to 3 minutes until smooth.
4. Serve and enjoy your Avocado Sauce!

Fragrant Tomato Sauce

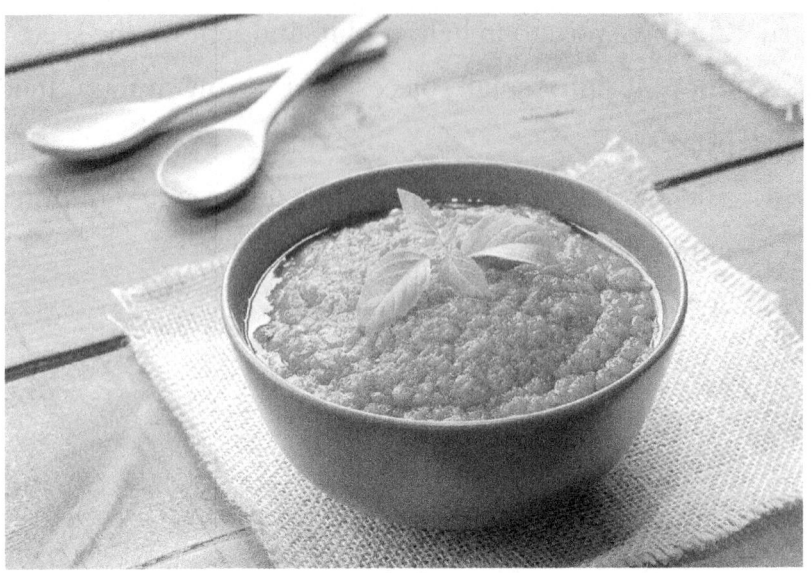

Cooking Time: 10 Minutes

Serving Size: 1 Cup

Ingredients

- 5 Roma Tomatoes
- 1 pinch of Basil
- 1 teaspoon of Oregano
- 1 teaspoon of Onion Powder
- 2 tablespoons of minced Onion
- 2 tablespoons of Agave Syrup
- 1 teaspoon of Pure Sea Salt
- 2 tablespoons of Grape Seed Oil

Cooking Instructions

1. Make an X cut on the bottom of the Roma Tomatoes and place them into a pot of boiling water for just 1 minute.
2. Remove the Tomatoes from the water with a spoon and shock them, placing them in cold water for 30 seconds.
3. Take them out and immediately peel with your fingers or a knife.
4. Put all the ingredients into a blender or a food processor and blend for 1 minute until smooth.
5. Serve and enjoy your Fragrant Tomato Sauce!

"Cheese" Sauce

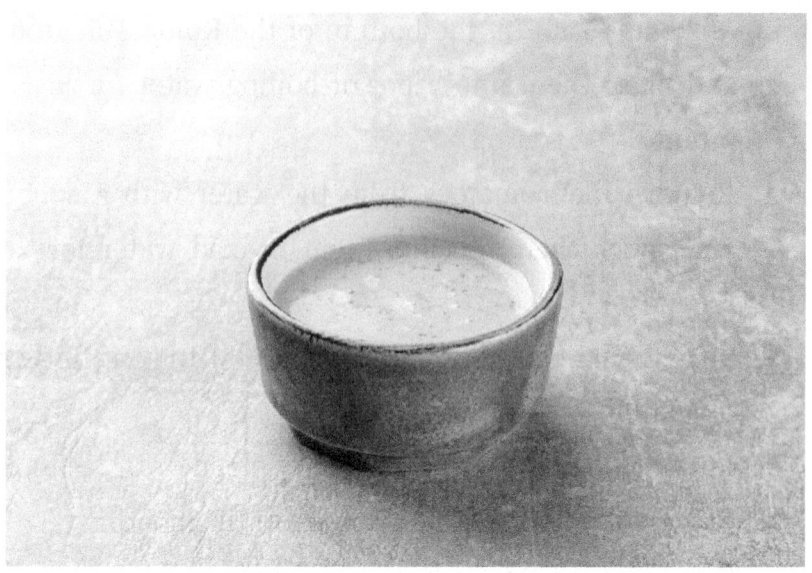

Cooking Time: 3 Hours 15 Minutes

Serving Size: 6 Cups

Ingredients

- 2 cups of Raw Brazil Nuts
- 1/2 teaspoon of Cayenne Powder
- 1 teaspoon of Onion Powder
- 2 teaspoons of Pure Sea Salt
- 1 1/2 cups of *Homemade Hempseed Milk (see recipe on page 132)*
- 2 tablespoons of Grape Seed Oil
- 1 1/2 cups of Spring Water

- Juice from a half of Lime

Cooking Instructions

1. Soak the Brazil Nuts overnight or for at least 3 hours. Pour out the water and rinse them.
2. Place all ingredients (using only 1/2 cup of the Spring Water) into a blender or a food processor.
3. Blend them together for about 2 minutes.
4. Add 1/2 cup of the Spring Water and blend it repeatedly.
5. Continue to add more water and blend the mixture until it attains a creamy consistency.
6. Allow to cool before serving.
7. Serve and enjoy your "Cheese" Sauce!

Guacamole

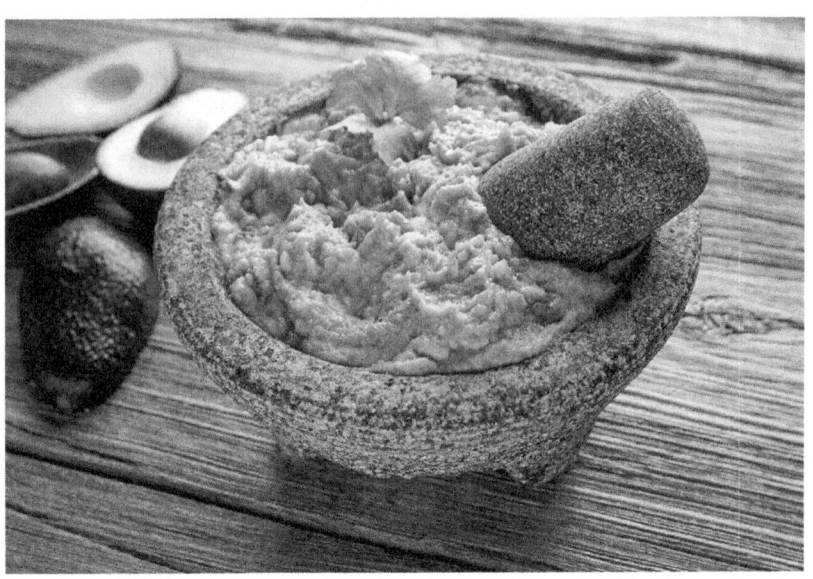

Cooking Time: 15 Minutes

Serving Size: 2 Cups

Ingredients
- 1 minced Roma Tomato
- 2 Avocados
- 1/2 cup of chopped Cilantro
- 1/2 cup of minced Red Onion
- 1/2 teaspoon of Cayenne Powder
- 1/2 teaspoon of Onion Powder
- 1/2 teaspoon of Pure Sea Salt
- Juice from a half of Lime

Cooking Instructions

1. Cut the Avocados in half, peel, and remove the seeds.
2. Chop into small pieces and put them in a medium bowl.
3. Add all other ingredients, excluding the Roma Tomato, to the bowl.
4. Using a masher, mix together until smooth.
5. Add the minced Roma Tomato to the mixture and mix well.
6. Serve* and enjoy your delicious Guacamole!

Useful Tips

*You can serve Guacamole with our *Flatbread (see recipe on page 146)* or *Tortilla Chips (see recipe on page 152)*.

"Garlic" Sauce

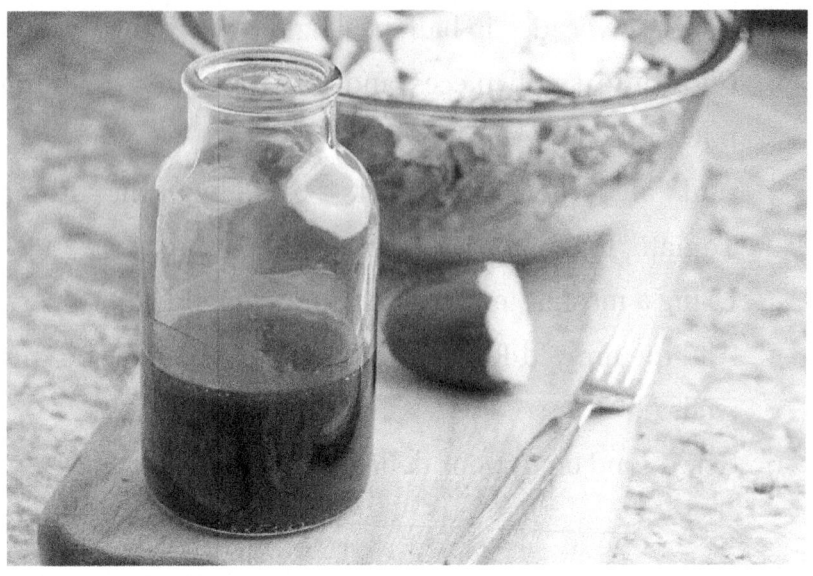

Cooking Time: 1 Hour 10 Minutes

Serving Size: 1 Cup

Ingredients

- 1/4 cup of diced Shallots
- 1 tablespoon of Onion Powder
- 1/4 teaspoon of Dill
- 1/2 teaspoon of Ginger
- 1/2 teaspoon of Pure Sea Salt
- 1 cup of Grape Seed Oil

Cooking Instructions

1. Find a glass jar with a lid.
2. Put all ingredients for the sauce in the jar and shake them well.
3. Place the sauce mixture in the refrigerator for at least 1 hour.
4. Serve and enjoy your "Garlic" Sauce!

Useful Tips

You can use this "Garlic" Sauce within 2 weeks. Store it in a glass jar with a lid in the refrigerator.

If you have a hand blender, mix all ingredients together. The sauce is prepared and you can use it immediately.

Olivia Shields

SPECIAL INGREDIENTS

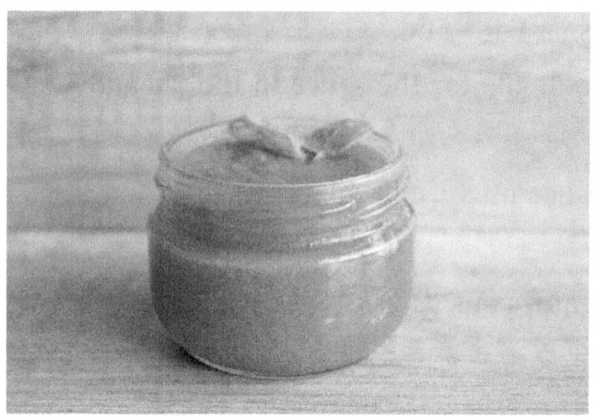

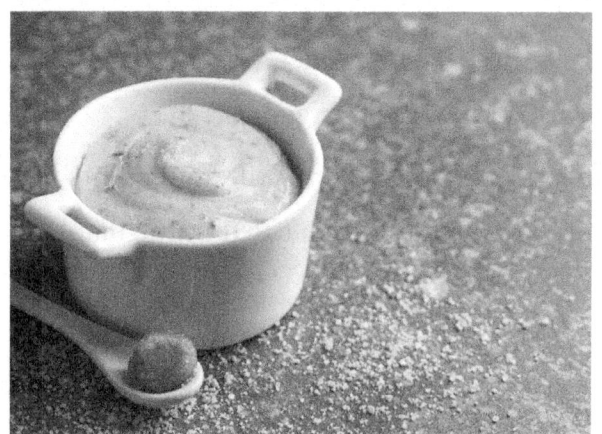

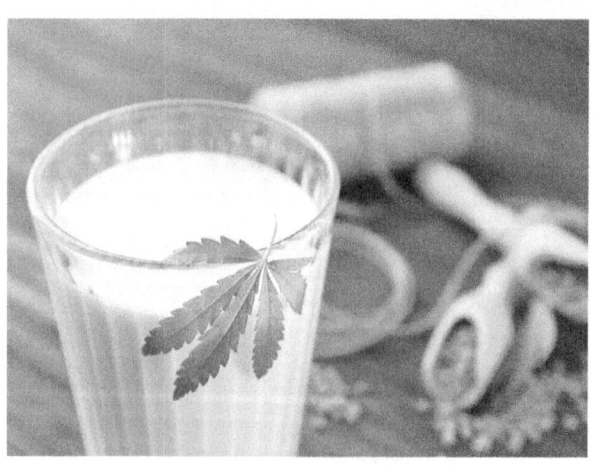

Spicy Infused Oil

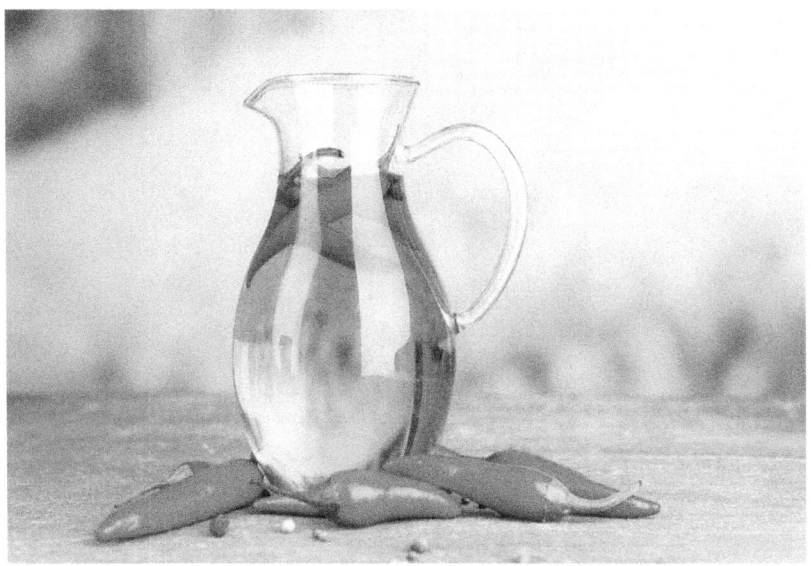

Cooking Time: 24 Hours

Serving Size: 1 Cup

Ingredients
- 1 tablespoon of crushed Cayenne Pepper
- 3/4 cup of Grape Seed Oil

Cooking Instructions
1. Fill a glass jar with a lid or a squeeze bottle with Grape Seed Oil.
2. Add crushed Cayenne Pepper to the jar/bottle.
3. Shake it and let the oil infuse for at least 24 hours.
4. Add it to a dish and enjoy your Spicy Infused Oil!

Homemade Walnut Milk

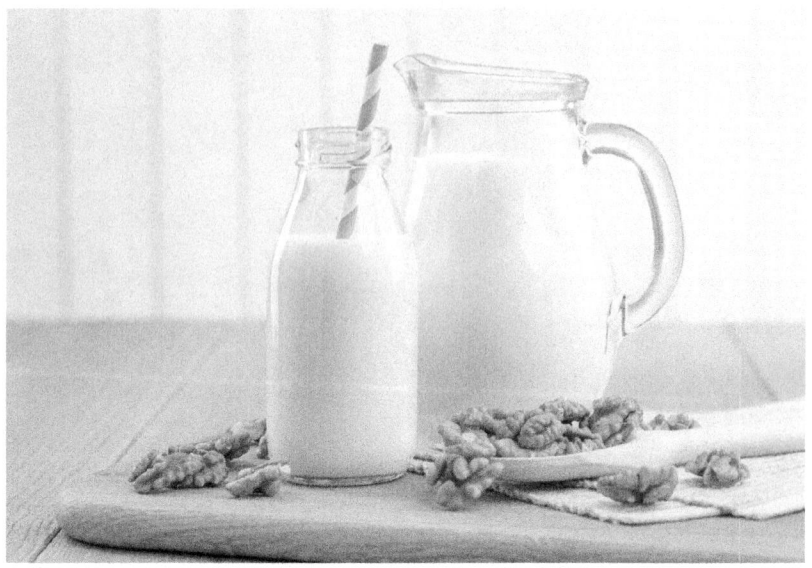

Cooking Time: Minimum 8 Hours

Serving Size: 4 Cups

Ingredients
- 1 cup of Raw Walnuts
- 1/8 teaspoon of Pure Sea Salt
- 3 cups of Spring Water + extra for soaking

Cooking Instructions
1. Put raw Walnuts in a small pot and cover them with three inches of water.
2. Soak the Walnuts for at least eight hours.
3. Drain and rinse the Walnuts with cold water.
4. Add the soaked Walnuts, Pure sea salt, and three cups of Spring Water to a blender.
5. Mix well until smooth.
6. Strain it if you need to.
7. Enjoy your Homemade Walnut Milk!

"Garlic" Infused Oil

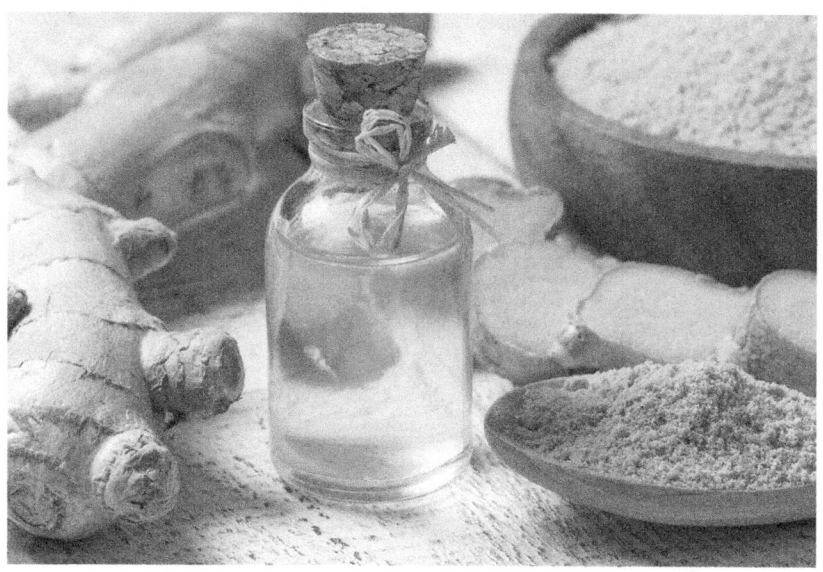

Cooking Time: 24 Hours

Serving Size: 1 Cup

Ingredients
- 1/2 teaspoon of Dill
- 1/2 teaspoon of Ginger Powder
- 1 tablespoon of Onion Powder
- 1/2 teaspoon of Pure Sea Salt
- 3/4 cup of Grape Seed Oil

Cooking Instructions
1. Fill a glass jar with a lid or a squeeze bottle with Grape Seed Oil.
2. Add the seasonings to the jar/bottle.
3. Shake it and let the oil infuse for at least 24 hours.
4. Add it to a dish and enjoy your "Garlic" Infused Oil!

Aquafaba

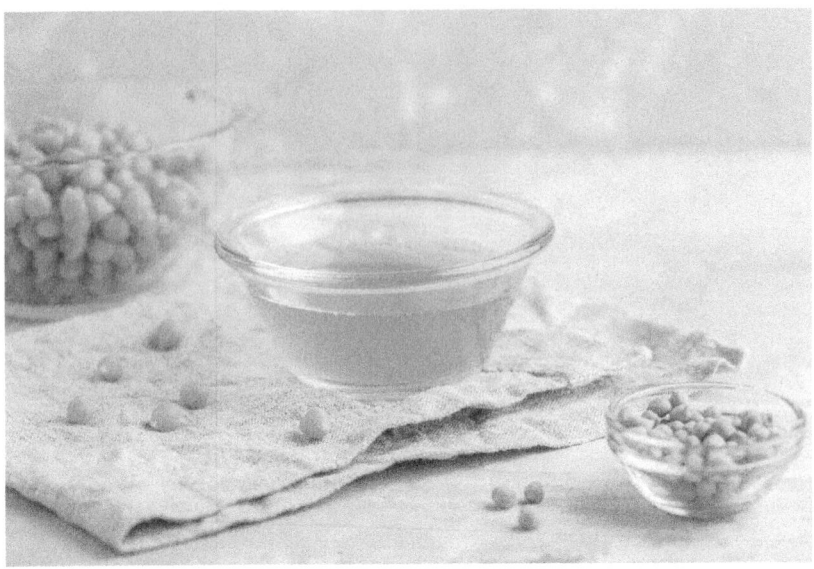

Cooking Time: 2 Hours 30 Minutes

Serving Size: 2-4 Cups

Ingredients
- 1 bag of Garbanzo Beans
- 1 teaspoon of Pure Sea Salt
- 6 cups of Spring Water + extra for soaking

Cooking Instructions
1. Place Garbanzo Beans in a large pot, add Spring Water and Pure Sea Salt. Bring to a rolling boil.
2. Remove from the heat and leave to soak for 30 to 40 minutes.

3. Strain Garbanzo Beans and add 6 cups of Spring Water.
4. Boil for 1 hour and 30 minutes on medium heat.
5. Strain the Garbanzo Beans. This strained water is Aquafaba.
6. Pour Aquafaba into a glass jar with a lid and place it into the refrigerator.
7. After cooling, Aquafaba becomes thicker. If it is too liquid, repeatedly boil for 10-20 minutes.

Useful Tips

Aquafaba is a good alternative for an egg:
- 2 tablespoons of *Aquafaba* = 1 egg white;
- 3 tablespoons of *Aquafaba* = 1 egg.

Homemade Hempseed Milk

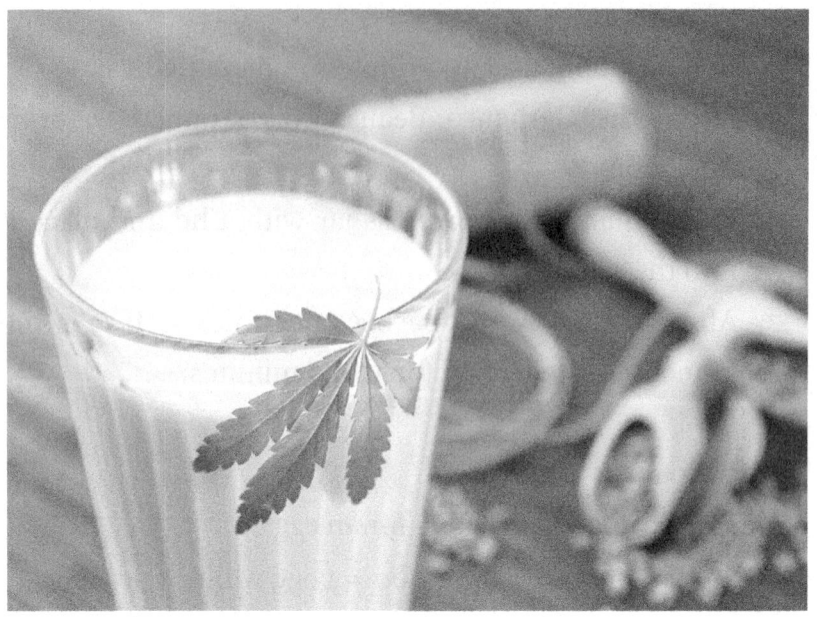

Cooking Time: 2 Hours

Serving Size: 2 Cups

Ingredients

- 2 tablespoons of Hemp Seeds
- 2 tablespoons of Agave Syrup
- 1/8 teaspoon of Pure Sea Salt
- 2 cups of Spring Water
- Fruits *(optional)**

Cooking Instructions

1. Place all ingredients, except fruits, into the blender.
2. Blend them for two minutes.
3. Add fruits and repeatedly blend for 30 to 50 seconds.
4. Leave milk in a refrigerator until cold.
5. Enjoy your Homemade Hempseed Milk!

Useful Tips

*You can add Blueberries, Baby Bananas, or other fruits from Doctor Sebi's approved food list to the milk.

Homemade Hempseed Milk can be kept in a refrigerator for up to 5 days. However, if you add fruits to the milk, it will only be fresh for 24 hours.

Olivia Shields

Papaya Seed Mango Dressing

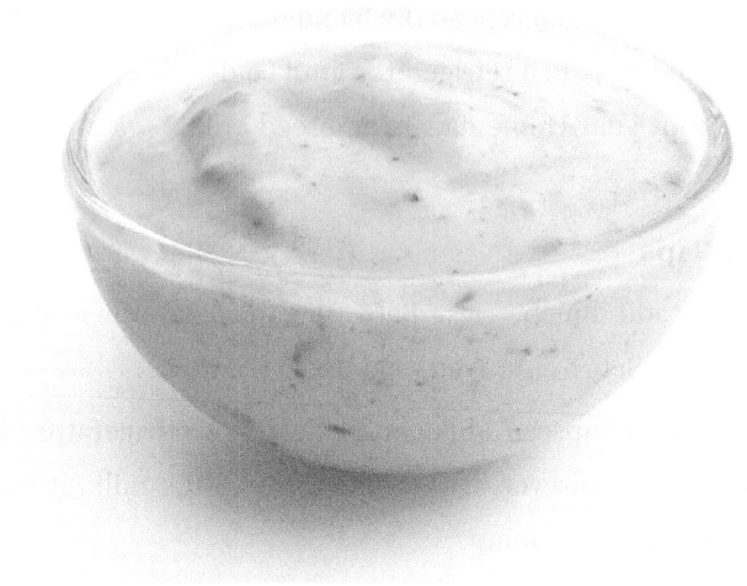

Cooking Time: 10 Minutes

Serving Size: 1/2 Cup

Ingredients

- 1 cup of chopped Mango
- 1 teaspoon of Ground Papaya Seeds
- 1 teaspoon of Basil
- 1 teaspoon of Onion Powder
- 1 teaspoon of Agave Syrup

- 2 tablespoons of Lime Juice
- 1/4 cup of Grape Seed Oil
- 1/4 teaspoon of Pure Sea Salt

Cooking Instructions

1. Prepare and place all ingredients into the blender.
2. Blend for one minute until smooth.
3. Add it to a salad and enjoy your Papaya Seed Mango Dressing!

Useful Tips

Seasonings can be altered according to your liking.

Use this dressing within two days. Store it in a sealed glass jar in the refrigerator.

Tomato Ginger Dressing

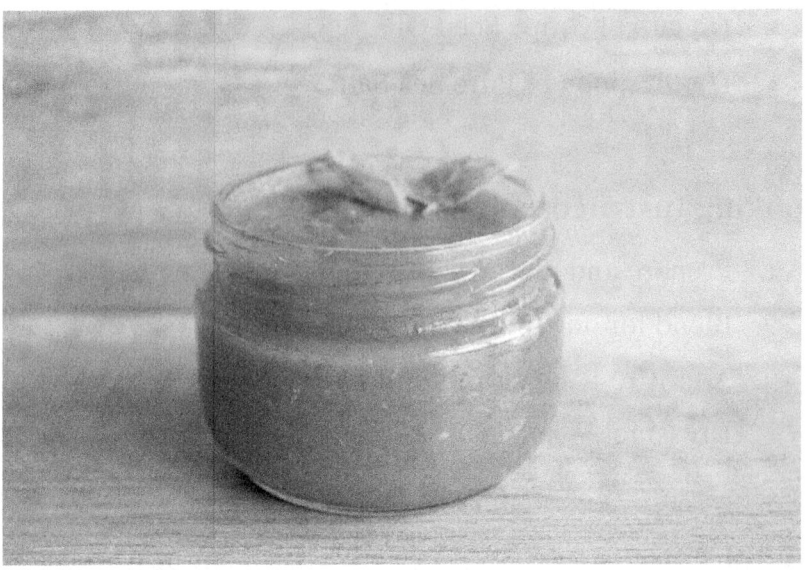

Cooking Time: 10 Minutes

Serving Size: 1/2 Cup

Ingredients

- 2 chopped Plum Tomatoes
- 1 teaspoon of minced Ginger*
- 1 tablespoon of Agave Syrup
- 2 tablespoons of chopped Onion
- 2 tablespoons of Sesame Seeds
- 1 tablespoon of Lime Juice

Cooking Instructions

1. Prepare and place all ingredients into the blender.
2. Blend for one minute until smooth.
3. Add it to a salad and enjoy your Tomato Ginger Dressing!

Useful Tips

*Remember, fresh ginger is much stronger than dried ginger.

Seasonings can be adjusted according to your liking.

Use this dressing within two days. Store it in a glass jar in the refrigerator.

Dill Cucumber Dressing

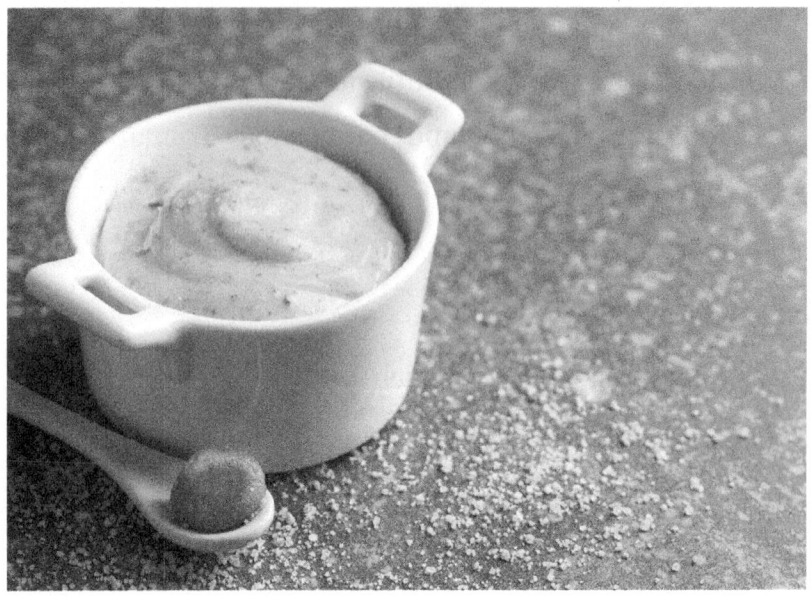

Cooking Time: 10 Minutes

Serving Size: 1/2 Cup

Ingredients

- 1 teaspoon of fresh Dill*
- 1 cup of quartered Cucumbers
- 1/2 teaspoon of Onion Powder
- 2 teaspoons of Agave Syrup
- 1 tablespoon of Lime Juice
- 1/4 cup of Avocado Oil

Cooking Instructions

1. Prepare and place all ingredients into the blender.
2. Blend for one minute until smooth.
3. Add it to a salad and enjoy your Dill Cucumber Dressing!

Useful Tips

*Remember, fresh dill is much stronger than dried dill.

Seasonings can be adjusted according to your liking.

Use this dressing within two days. Store it in a glass jar in the refrigerator.

Italian Infused Oil

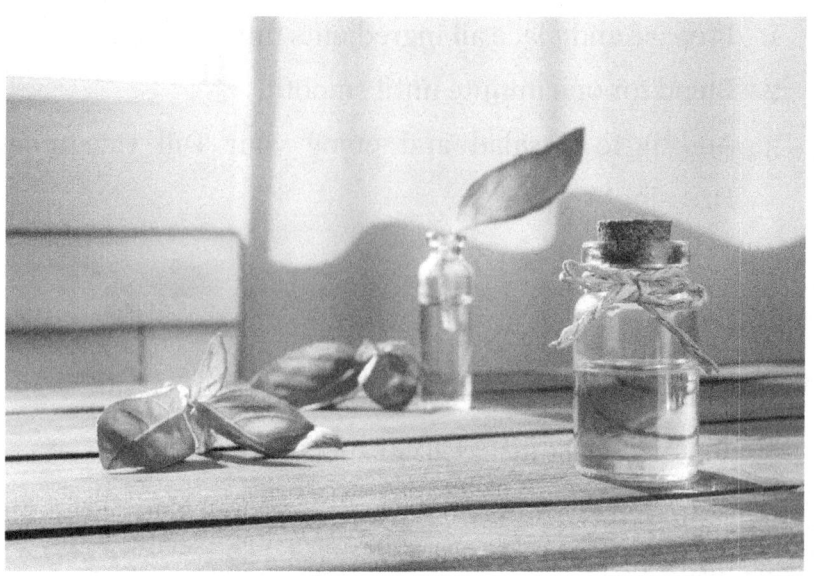

Cooking Time: 24 Hours

Serving Size: 1 Cup

Ingredients

- 1 teaspoon of Oregano
- 1 teaspoon of Basil
- 1 pinch of Pure Sea Salt
- 3/4 cup of Grape Seed Oil

Cooking Instructions

1. Fill a glass jar with a lid or a squeeze bottle with Grape Seed Oil.
2. Mix seasoning together and add them to the jar/bottle.
3. Shake it and let the oil infuse for at least 24 hours.
4. Add it to a dish and enjoy your Italian Infused Oil!

SNACKS & BREAD

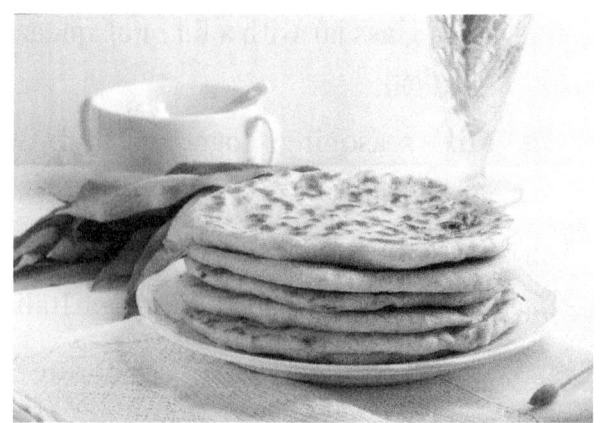

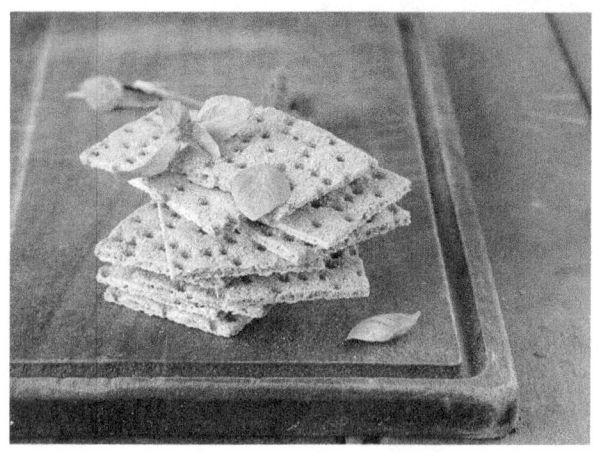

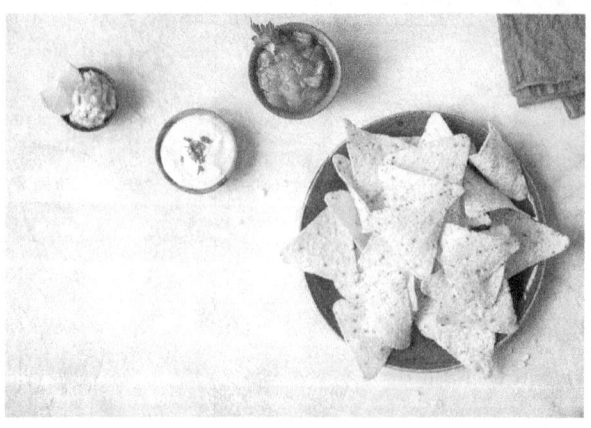

Onion Rings

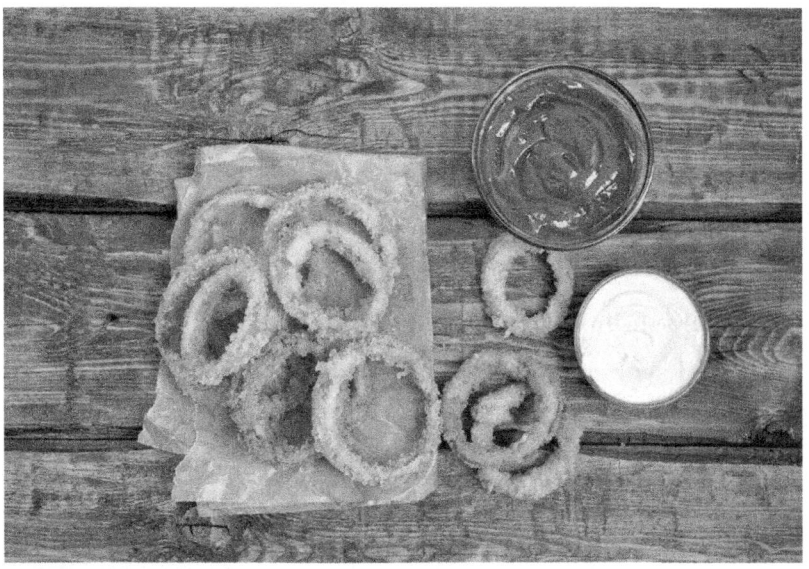

Cooking Time: 30 Minutes

Serving Size: 8 Servings

Ingredients

- White Onions or Sweet Onions
- 1 cup of Spelt Flour
- 1/2 cup of *Homemade Hempseed Milk (see recipe on page 132)*
- 1/2 cup of *Aquafaba (see recipe on page 130)*
- 2 teaspoons of Onion Powder
- 2 teaspoons of Oregano
- 1 teaspoon of Cayenne Powder

- 2 teaspoons of Pure Sea Salt
- 3 tablespoons of Grape Seed Oil

Cooking Instructions

1. Preheat your oven to 450 degrees Fahrenheit.
2. Pour *Homemade Hempseed Milk* and *Aquafaba* into a medium bowl and whisk them well.
3. Add 1 teaspoon of Oregano, 1 teaspoon of Onion Powder, 1/2 teaspoon of Cayenne, and 1 teaspoon of Pure Sea Salt to the wet ingredients and mix.
4. Peel the Onions, slice off the ends.
5. Cut the peeled onion into slices about 1/4 inch thick. Separate the onion slices into rings.
6. Add Spelt Flour, 1 teaspoon of Oregano, 1 teaspoon of Onion Powder, 1/2 teaspoon of Cayenne, and 1 teaspoon of Pure Sea Salt to a container with a lid. Shake all the dry ingredients well.
7. Brush a baking sheet with Grape Seed Oil
8. Place a few onion rings in the wet mixture.
9. Put wet onion rings in the dry mixture and flip until coated on both sides
10. Put the covered onion rings on the baking sheet.
11. Repeat steps 8 through 10 until all onion rings are covered.
12. Lightly drizzle the rings with Grape Seed Oil.
13. Bake for about 10 to 15 minutes until golden brown.

14. Allow to cool them before serving.
15. Serve and enjoy your Onion Rings!

Useful Tips

*If you don't have prepared *Aquafaba*, add just 1/2 more cup of *Homemade Hempseed Milk (see recipe on page 132)*.

You can serve Onion Rings with our *Sweet Barbecue Sauce (see recipe on page 114)*, or *"Cheese" Sauce (see recipe on page 120)*.

Flatbread

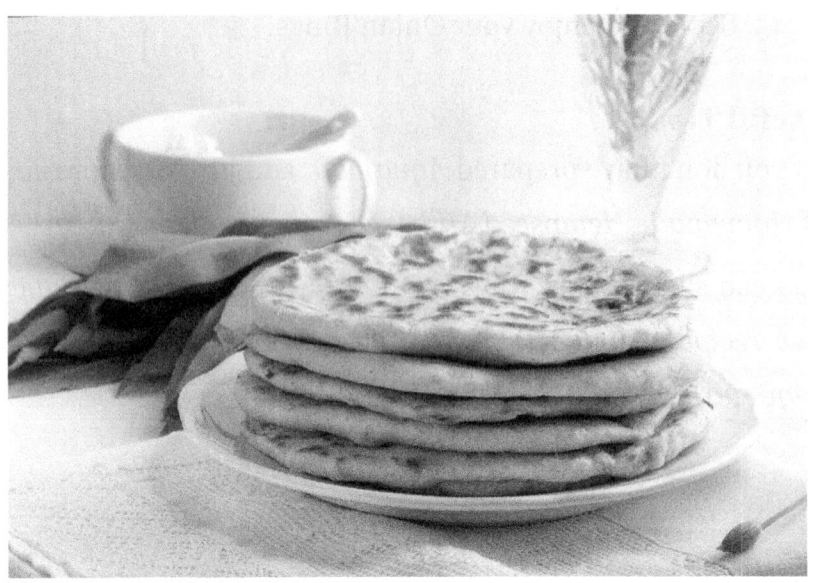

Cooking Time: 20 Minutes

Serving Size: 6 Servings

Ingredients

- 2 cups of Spelt Flour
- 2 teaspoons of Oregano
- 2 teaspoons of Onion Powder
- 1/4 teaspoon of Cayenne
- 2 teaspoons of Basil
- 1 tablespoon of Pure Sea Salt
- 3/4 cup of Spring Water
- 2 tablespoons of Grape Seed Oil

Cooking Instructions

1. Add the Spelt Flour and all seasonings into a medium bowl and mix them well.
2. Add the Grape Seed Oil and 1/2 cup of Spring Water and continue to mix.
3. Try to form the mixture into a dough ball. If it is too thick, add more Spring Water.
4. Prepare a place for rolling out the dough and cover it with flour.
5. Knead the dough for about 5 minutes until it achieves the desired consistency.
6. Divide the dough into 6 equal balls.
7. Roll out each ball into circles about 4 inches in diameter.
8. Heat a non-stick pan. Place one flatbread in the pan and cook on medium heat.
9. Flip the Flatbread every 2 to 3 minutes and cook until it is done. Small golden brown spots should appear on both sides.
10. Continue to cook the rest of the pieces.
11. Serve and enjoy your Flatbread!

Useful Tips

You can adjust seasonings according to your liking.

Healthy Crackers

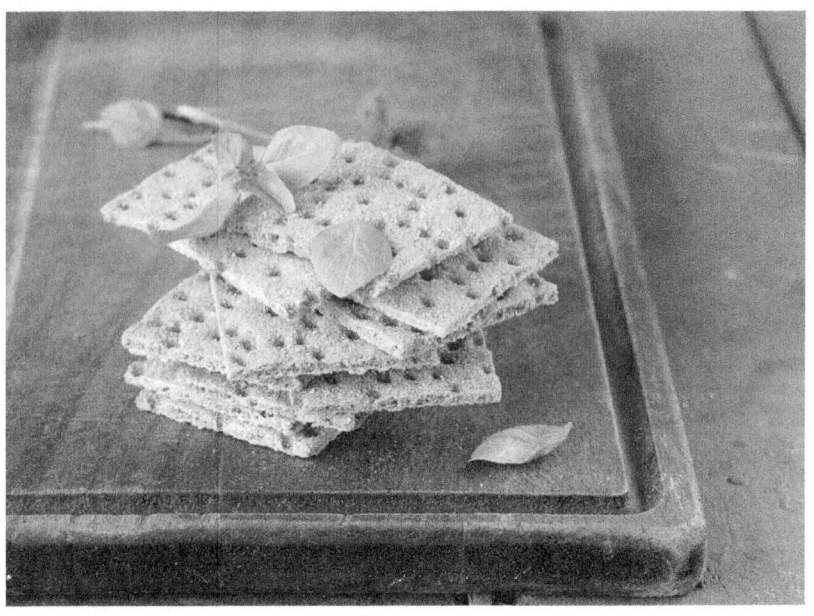

Cooking Time: 30 Minutes

Serving Size: 50 Crackers

Ingredients

- 1/2 cup of Rye Flour
- 1 cup of Spelt Flour
- 2 teaspoons of Sesame Seed
- 1 teaspoon of Agave Syrup
- 1 teaspoon of Pure Sea Salt
- 2 tablespoons of Grape Seed Oil
- 3/4 cup of Spring Water

Cooking Instructions

1. Preheat your oven to 350 degrees Fahrenheit.
2. Add all ingredients to a medium bowl and mix well.
3. Make a dough ball. If the consistency is too liquid, add more flour to it.
4. Prepare a place for rolling out the dough and cover it with a piece of parchment paper.
5. Lightly grease the paper with Grape Seed Oil and place the dough on it.
6. Roll out the dough with a rolling pin, adding more flour to avoid sticking.
7. When your dough is rolled out, take a shape cutter and cut the dough into squares. If you don't have a shape cutter, you can use a pizza cutter.
8. Place the squares on a baking pan and poke holes in each square using a fork or a skewer.
9. Brush the dough with a little Grape Seed Oil and sprinkle with more Pure Sea Salt if desired.
10. Bake for 12 to 15 minutes or until crackers are starting to become golden.
11. Allow to cool before serving.
12. Serve and enjoy your Healthy Crackers!

Useful Tips

You can add any seasonings from Doctor Sebi's food list according to your liking.

You can serve Crackers with our *Fragrant Tomato Sauce (see recipe on page 118), Avocado Sauce (see recipe on page 116)* or *"Cheese" Sauce (see recipe on page 120).*

Tortillas

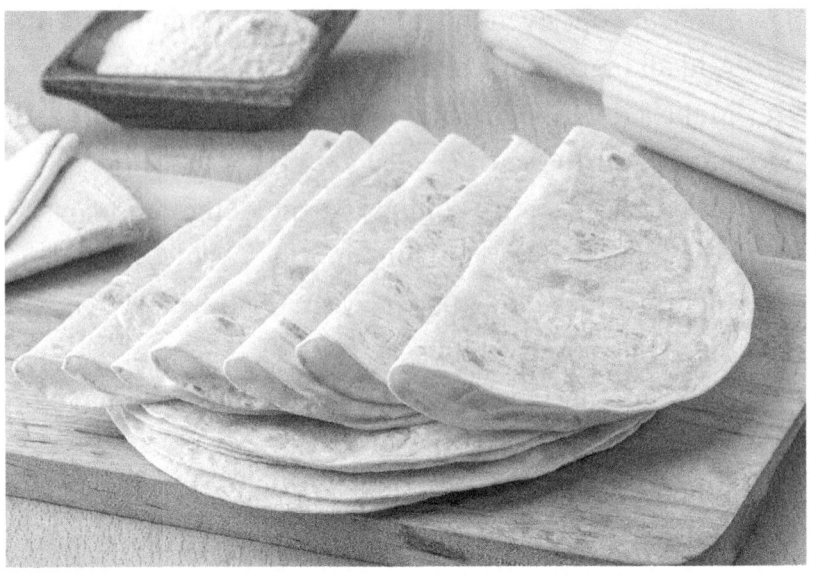

Cooking Time: 20 Minutes

Serving Size: 8 Servings

Ingredients

- 2 cups of Spelt Flour
- 1 teaspoon of Pure Sea Salt
- 1/2 cup of Spring Water

Cooking Instructions

1. Combine the Spelt Flour with Pure Sea Salt in a food processor*. Mix for about 15 seconds.

2. Continue blending, slowly add Grape Seed Oil until well incorporated.
3. Slowly add Spring Water while blending until a dough is formed.
4. Prepare a work surface and cover it with a piece of parchment paper. Sprinkle with flour.
5. Knead the dough for about 1 to 2 minutes until it achieves the right consistency.
6. Divide the dough into 8 equal balls.
7. Roll out each ball into a very thin circle.
8. Heat a non-stick pan, cook one tortilla at a time on medium heat for about 30 to 60 seconds on each side.
9. Serve and enjoy your Tortillas!

Useful Tips

*If you don't have a food processor, you can use a hand mixer or a blender. However, you will have better results with a food processor.

You can serve Tortillas with our *Sweet Barbecue Sauce (see recipe on page 114), Avocado Sauce (see recipe on page 116),* or *"Cheese" Sauce (see recipe on page 120).*

Tortilla Chips

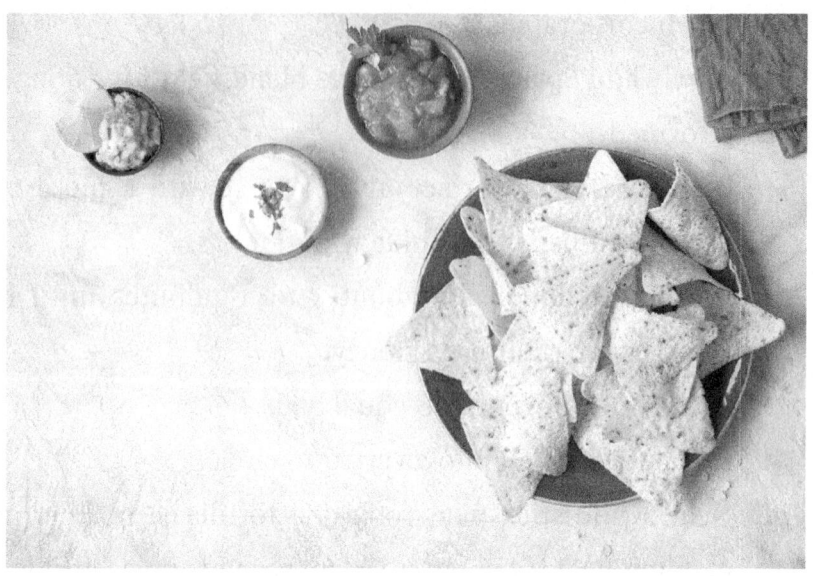

Cooking Time: 30 Minutes

Serving Size: 8 Servings

Ingredients

- 2 cups of Spelt Flour
- 1 teaspoon of Pure Sea Salt
- 1/2 cup of Spring Water
- 1/3 cup of Grape Seed Oil

Cooking Instructions

1. Preheat your oven to 350 degrees Fahrenheit.

2. Combine the Spelt Flour with Pure Sea Salt in a food processor*. Mix for about 15 seconds.
3. While blending, slowly add Grape Seed Oil until it is well combined.
4. Continue to blend and slowly add Spring Water until a dough is formed.
5. Prepare a work surface and cover it with a piece of parchment paper. Sprinkle flour over the paper.
6. Knead the dough for about 1 to 2 minutes until it achieves the right consistency.
7. Cover a baking pan with a little Grape Seed Oil.
8. Put the prepared dough on the baking pan.
9. Brush dough with a little Grape Seed Oil and sprinkle with more Pure Sea Salt if desired.
10. Cut the dough into 8 triangles with a pizza slicer.
11. Bake for about 10 to 12 minutes or until the chips are starting to become golden brown.
12. Allow to cool before serving.
13. Serve and enjoy your Tortilla Chips!

Useful Tips

*If you don't have a food processor, you can use a hand mixer or a blender. However, you will receive better results with a food processor.

You can serve Tortillas with our *Sweet Barbecue Sauce (see recipe on page 114), Guacamole (see recipe on page 122),* or *"Cheese" Sauce (see recipe on page 120).*

DESSERTS

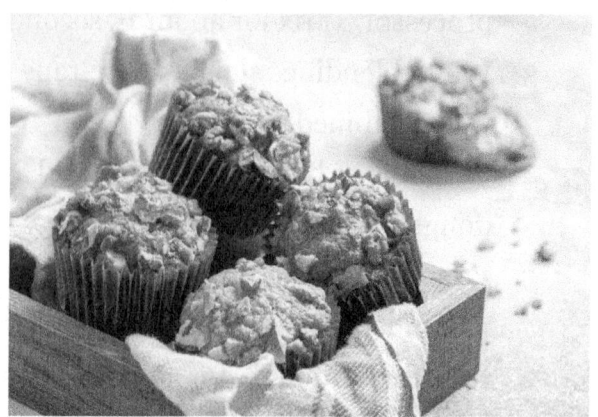

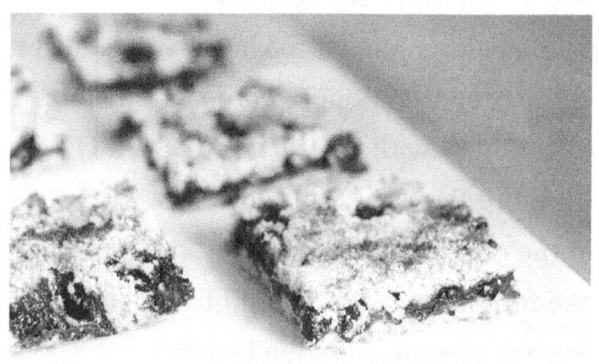

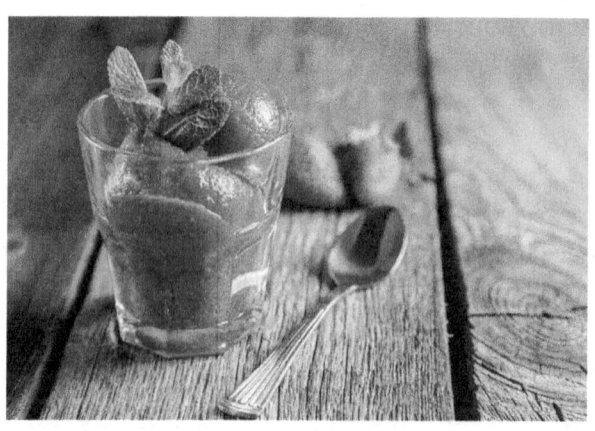

Squash Pie

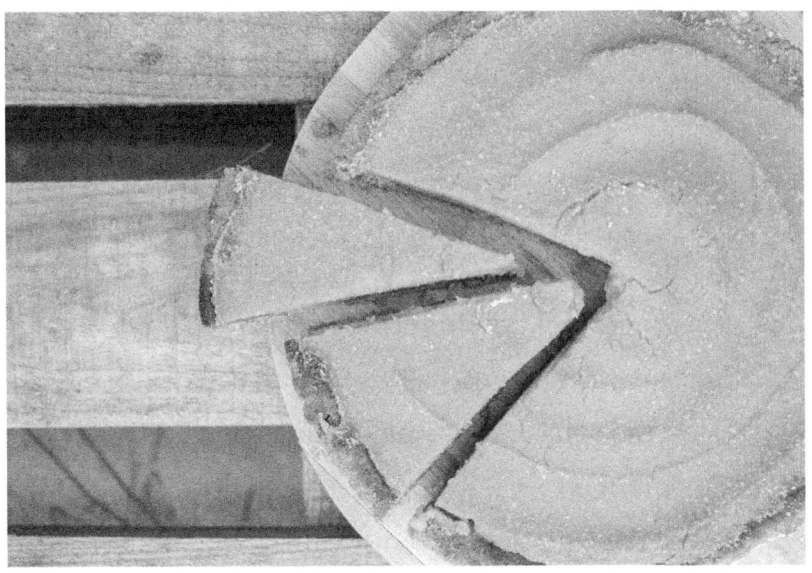

Cooking Time: 2 Hour 30 Minutes

Serving Size: 6-8 Servings

Ingredients

- 2 Butternut Squashes
- 1 1/4 cups of Spelt Flour
- 1/4 cup of Date Sugar
- 1/4 cup of Agave Syrup
- 1 teaspoon of Allspice
- 1 teaspoon of Pure Sea Salt
- 1/4 cup of Spring Water

- 1/3 cup of Grape Seed Oil
- 1/4 cup of *Homemade Hempseed Milk (see recipe on page 132)**

Cooking Instructions

Filling:

1. Rinse and peel the Butternut Squashes.
2. Cut them in half and use a spoon to de-seed.
3. Chop the squash into small chunks and add them into a medium pot.
4. Cover the squash in Spring Water and boil it for 20 to 25 minutes until cooked.
5. Pour out the water and mash the cooked squash.
6. Add Date Sugar, Agave Syrup, 1/8 teaspoon of Pure Sea Salt, and *Homemade Hempseed Milk* and mix them thoroughly.

Crust:

7. Preheat your oven to 350 degrees Fahrenheit.
8. In a bowl, add Spelt Flour, 1/2 teaspoon of Pure Sea Salt, Spring Water, and Grape Seed Oil and mix.
9. Knead dough into a ball. Add more water or flour as needed. Allow it to rest for 5 minutes.
10. Spread out Spelt Flour on a piece of parchment paper.

11. Roll out the dough on the paper by rolling pin, adding more flour to avoid sticking.
12. Place the dough into a pie plate and bake it in the oven for 10 minutes.
13. Remove the crust from the oven, add the pie filling, and bake for another 40 minutes.
14. Remove the pie and leave it for 30 minutes until cool.
15. Serve and enjoy your Squash Pie!

Useful Tips

*If you don't have *Homemade Hempseed Milk*, you can substitute *Homemade Walnut Milk (see recipe on page 128).*

Strawberry Sorbet

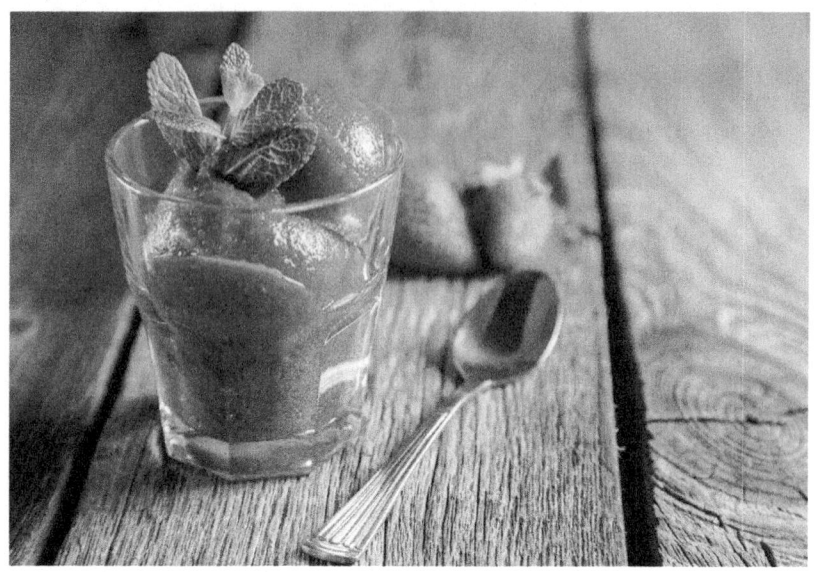

Cooking Time: 4 Hours

Serving Size: 4 Servings

Ingredients
- 2 cups of Strawberries*
- 1 1/2 teaspoons of Spelt Flour
- 1/2 cup of Date Sugar
- 2 cups of Spring Water

Cooking Instructions
1. Add Date Sugar, Spring Water, and Spelt Flour to a medium pot and boil on low heat for about ten minutes. Mixture should thicken, like syrup.

2. Remove the pot from the heat and allow it to cool.
3. After cooling, add pureed Strawberry and mix gently.
4. Put this mixture in a container and freeze.
5. Cut it into pieces, put the sorbet into a processor and blend until smooth.
6. Put everything back in the container and leave in the refrigerator for at least four hours.
7. Serve and enjoy your Strawberry Sorbet!

Useful Tips

*If you don't have fresh berries, you can use frozen ones.

Blueberry Muffins

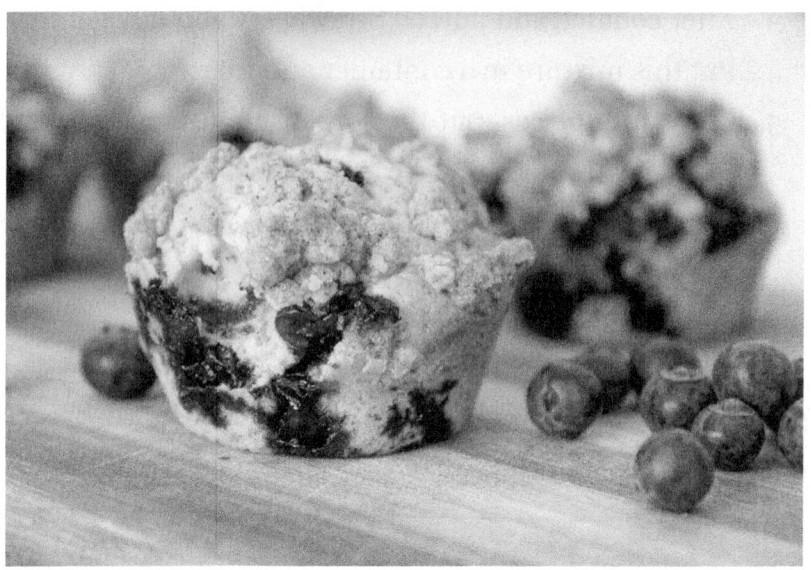

Cooking Time: 1 Hour

Serving Size: 3 Servings

Ingredients
- 1/2 cup of Blueberries
- 3/4 cup of Teff Flour
- 3/4 cup of Spelt Flour
- 1/3 cup of Agave Syrup
- 1/2 teaspoon of Pure Sea Salt
- 1 cup of Coconut Milk
- 1/4 cup of Sea Moss Gel *(optional, check information on page 18)*
- Grape Seed Oil

Cooking Instructions

1. Preheat your oven to 365 degrees Fahrenheit.
2. Grease or line 6 standard muffin cups.
3. Add Teff, Spelt flour, Pure Sea Salt, Coconut Milk, Sea Moss Gel, and Agave Syrup to a large bowl. Mix them together.
4. Add Blueberries to the mixture and mix well.
5. Divide muffin batter among the 6 muffin cups.
6. Bake for 30 minutes until golden brown.
7. Serve and enjoy your Blueberry Muffins!

Banana Strawberry Ice Cream

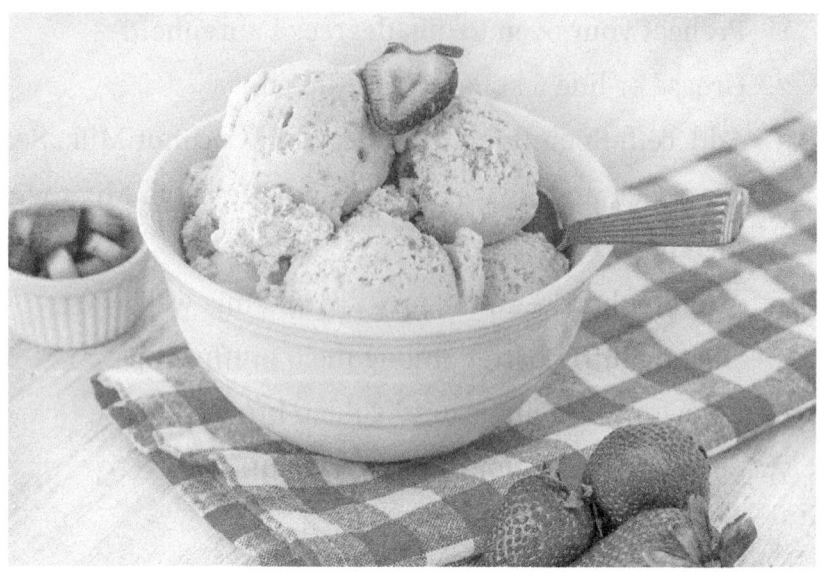

Cooking Time: 4 Hours

Serving Size: 5 Servings

Ingredients

- 1 cup of Strawberry*
- 5 quartered Baby Bananas*
- 1/2 Avocado, chopped
- 1 tablespoon of Agave Syrup
- 1/4 cup of *Homemade Walnut Milk (see recipe on page 128)***

Cooking Instructions

1. Put all ingredients into the blender and blend them well.
2. Taste. If it is too thick, add extra Milk or Agave Syrup if you want it sweeter.
3. Place in a container with a lid and allow to freeze for at least 5 to 6 hours.
4. Serve it and enjoy your Banana Strawberry Ice Cream!

Useful Tips

*If you don't have fresh berries or bananas, you can use frozen ones.

You can use any fruits you wish but be sure to use avocado every time. The fat in Avocado helps to make a creamier consistency.

**If you don't have *Homemade Walnut Milk,* you can substitute *Homemade Hempseed Milk (see recipe on page 132).*

Homemade Whipped Cream

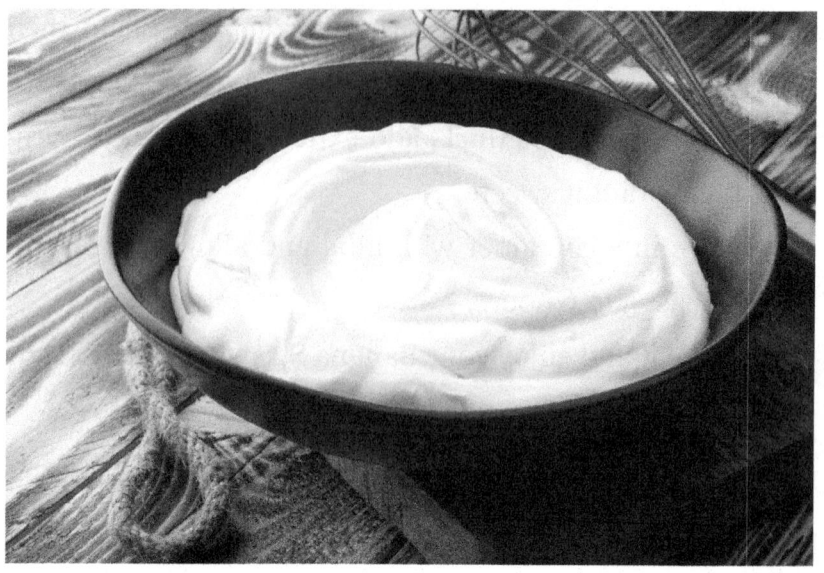

Cooking Time: 10 Minutes

Serving Size: 1 Cup

Ingredients

- 1 cup of *Aquafaba (see recipe on page 130)*
- 1/4 cup of Agave Syrup

Cooking Instructions

1. Add Agave Syrup and *Aquafaba* into a bowl.
2. Mix at high speed around 5 minutes with a stand mixer or 10 to 15 minutes with a hand mixer.

3. Serve and enjoy your Homemade Whipped Cream!

Useful Tips

Store in the refrigerator if you don't use it immediately.

Whipped Cream will turn back to *Aquafaba* consistency eventually, just whip it again until thick.

"Chocolate" Pudding

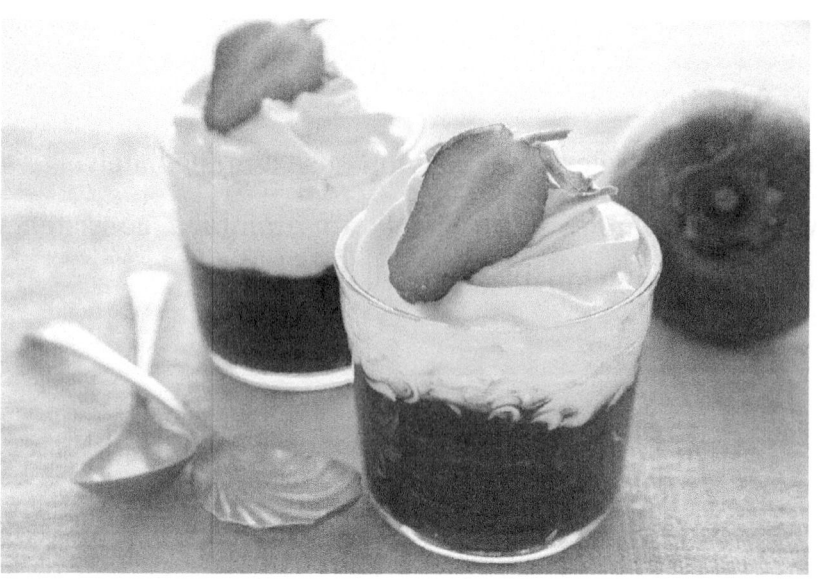

Cooking Time: 20 Minutes

Serving Size: 4 Servings

Ingredients

- 1 to 2 cups of Black Sapote
- 1/4 cup of Agave Syrup
- 1/2 cup of soaked Brazil Nuts (overnight or for at least 3 hours)
- 1 tablespoon of Hemp Seeds
- 1/2 cup of Spring Water

Cooking Instructions

1. Cut 1 to 2 cups of Black Sapote in half.
2. Remove all seeds. You should have 1 full cup of de-seeded fruit.
3. Put all ingredients into a blender and blend until smooth.
4. Serve and enjoy your "Chocolate" Pudding!

Useful Tips

Store in the refrigerator if you don't use immediately.

You can serve it with our *Homemade Whipped Cream (see recipe on page 164)*.

Banana Nut Muffins

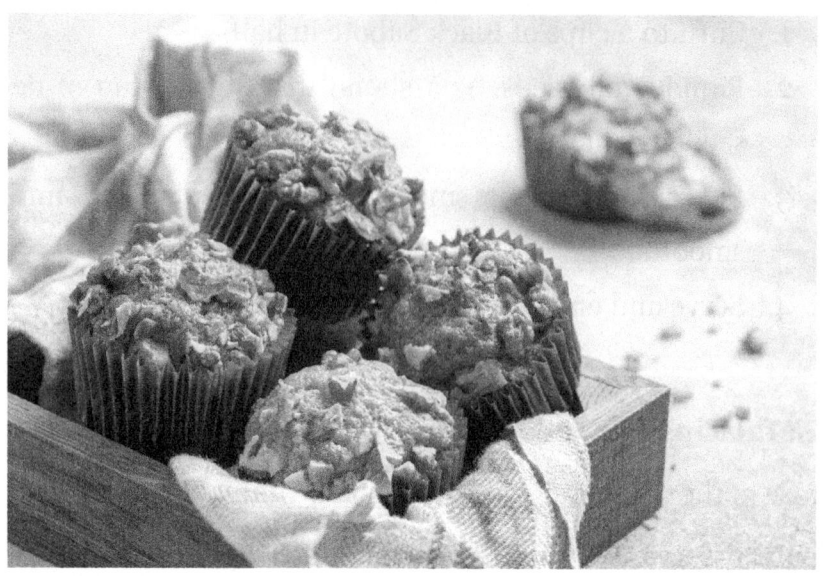

Cooking Time: 1 Hour

Serving Size: 6 Servings

Ingredients

Dry ingredients:
- 1 1/2 cups of Spell or Teff Flour
- 1/2 teaspoon of Pure Sea Salt
- 3/4 cup of Date Syrup

Wet ingredients:
- 2 medium pureed Burro Bananas
- ¼ cup of Grape Seed Oil
- ¾ cup of *Homemade Walnut Milk (see recipe on page 128)*

- 1 tablespoon of Key Lime Juice

Filling ingredients:
- ½ cup of chopped Walnuts (plus extra for decorating)
- 1 chopped Burro Banana

Cooking Instructions
1. Preheat your oven to 400 degrees Fahrenheit.
2. Take a muffin tray and grease 12 cups or line with cupcake liners.
3. Put all dry ingredients in a large bowl and mix them thoroughly.
4. Add all wet ingredients to a separate, smaller bowl and mix well with pureed Bananas.
5. Mix ingredients from the two bowls in one large container. Be careful not to over mix.
6. Add the filling ingredients and fold in gently.
7. Pour muffin batter into the 12 prepared muffin cups and garnish with a couple Walnuts.
8. Bake for 22 to 26 minutes until golden brown.
9. Allow to cool for 10 minutes.
10. Serve and enjoy your Banana Nut Muffins!

Useful Tips

*If you don't have *Homemade Walnut Milk,* you can substitute *Homemade Hempseed Milk (see recipe on page 132)*.

Mango Nut Cheesecake

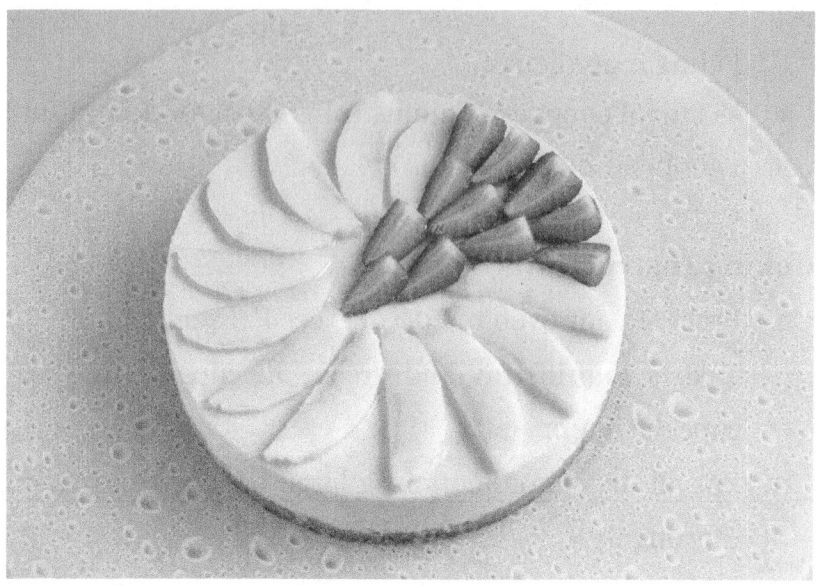

Cooking Time: 4 Hour 30 Minutes

Serving Size: 8 Servings

Ingredients

Filling:
- 2 cups of Brazil Nuts
- 5 to 6 Dates
- 1 tablespoon of Sea Moss Gel *(check information on page 18)*
- 1/4 cup of Agave Syrup
- 1/4 teaspoon of Pure Sea Salt
- 2 tablespoons of Lime Juice
- 1 1/2 cups of *Homemade Walnut Milk (see recipe on page 128)*

Crust:
- 1 1/2 cups of quartered Dates
- 1/4 cup of Agave Syrup
- 1 1/2 cups of Coconut Flakes
- 1/4 teaspoon of Pure Sea Salt

Toppings:
- Sliced Mango
- Sliced Strawberries

Cooking Instructions
1. Put all crust ingredients in a food processor and blend for 30 seconds.
2. Cover a baking form with parchment paper and spread out the blended crust ingredients.
3. Put sliced Mango across the crust and freeze for 10 minutes.
4. Blend all filling ingredients in a blender until smooth.
5. Pour the filling over the crust, cover with foil or parchment paper and let it stand for 3 to 4 hours in the refrigerator.
6. Take out from the baking form and garnish with toppings.
7. Serve and enjoy your Mango Nut Cheesecake!

Useful Tips
*If you don't have *Homemade Walnut Milk*, you can substitute *Homemade Hempseed Milk (see recipe on page 132)*.

Blackberry Jam

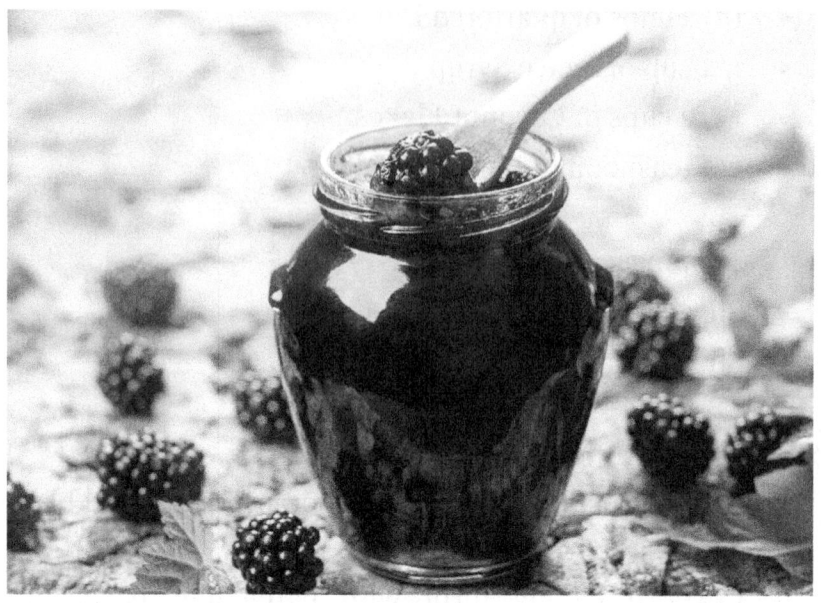

Cooking Time: 4 Hour 30 Minutes

Serving Size: 1 Cup

Ingredients

- 3/4 cup of Blackberries
- 1 tablespoon of Key Lime Juice
- 3 tablespoons of Agave Syrup
- ¼ cup of Sea Moss Gel + extra 2 tablespoons *(check information on page 18)*

Cooking Instructions

1. Put rinsed Blackberries into a medium pot and cook on medium heat.
2. Stir Blackberries until liquid appears.
3. Once berries soften, use your immersion blender to chop up any large pieces. If you don't have a blender put the mixture in a food processor, mix it well, then return to the pot.
4. Add Sea Moss Gel, Key Lime Juice and Agave Syrup to the blended mixture. Boil on medium heat and stir well until it becomes thick.
5. Remove from the heat and leave it to cool for 10 minutes.
6. Serve it with bread pieces or the *Flatbread (see recipe on page 146)*.
7. Enjoy your Blackberry Jam!

Useful Tips

*If you don't have Sea Moss Gel, you can omit it. However, the gel gives the jam a thicker consistency. Blackberries have natural pectin, which can achieve a similar effect.

Store this Blackberry Jam in a mason jar with a lid in the refrigerator for 2 to 3 weeks.

Don't store at room temperature!

Blackberry Bars

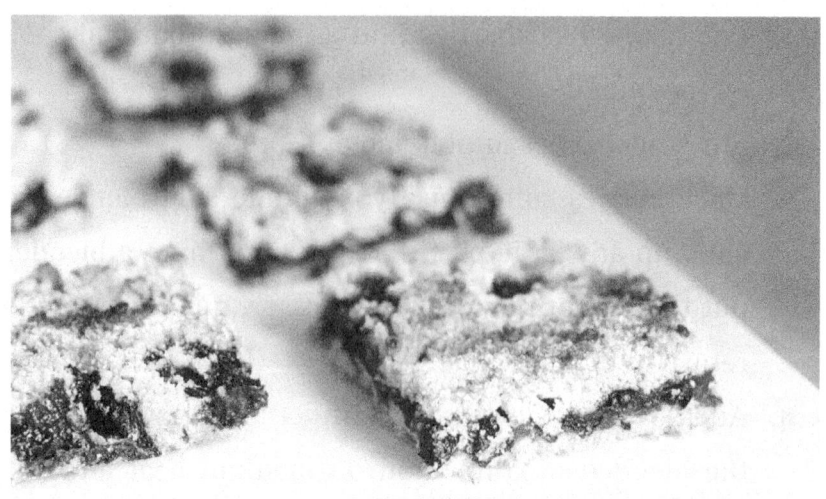

Cooking Time: 1 Hour 20 Minutes

Serving Size: 4 Servings

Ingredients

- 3 Burro Bananas or 4 Baby Bananas
- 1 cup of Spelt Flour
- 2 cups of Quinoa Flakes
- 1/4 cup of Agave Syrup
- 1/4 teaspoon of Pure Sea Salt
- 1/2 cup of Grape Seed Oil
- 1 cup of prepared *Blackberry Jam (see recipe on page 172).*

Cooking Instructions

1. Preheat your oven to 350 degrees Fahrenheit.
2. Peel Bananas and mash with a fork in a large bowl.
3. Combine Agave Syrup and Grape Seed Oil with the puree and mix well.
4. Add Spelt Flour and Quinoa Flakes. Knead the dough until it becomes sticky to your fingers.
5. Cover a 9x9-inch baking pan with parchment paper.
6. Take 2/3 of the dough and smooth it out over the parchment pan with your fingers.
7. Spread *Blackberry Jam* over the dough.
8. Crumble the remainder dough and sprinkle on the top.
9. Bake for 20 minutes.
10. Remove from the oven and let it cool for at 10 to 15 minutes.
11. Cut into small pieces.
12. Serve and enjoy your Blackberry Bars!

Useful Tips

You can keep this Blackberry Bar in the refrigerator for 5 to 6 days or in the freezer up to 3 months.

SMOOTHIES

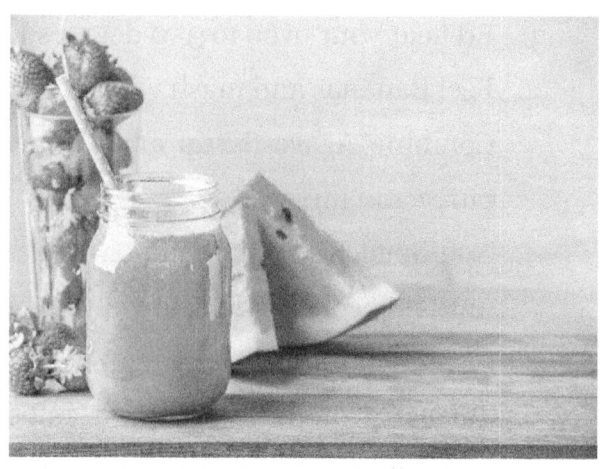

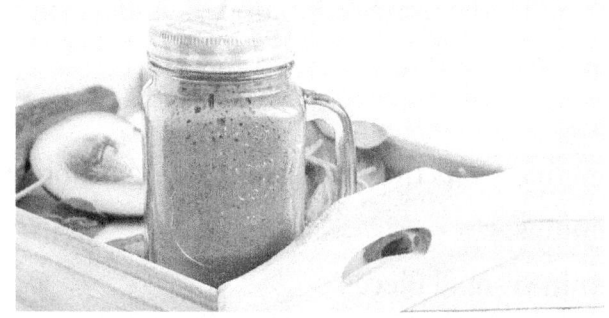

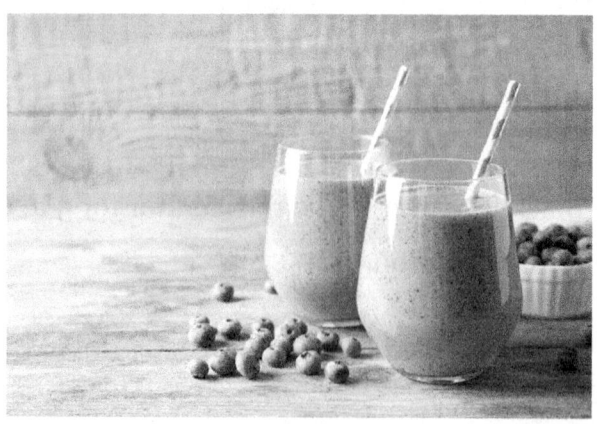

Creamy Mango Smoothie

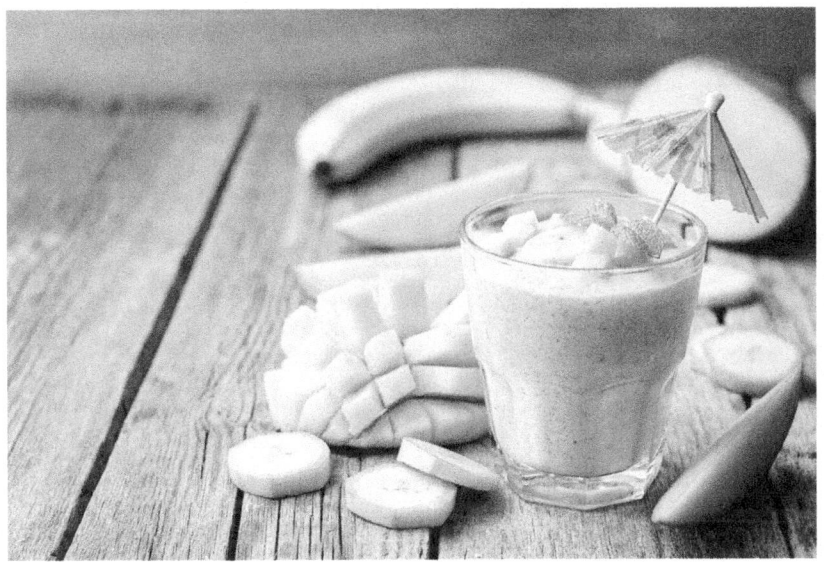

Cooking Time: 10 Minutes

Serving Size: 2 Servings

Ingredients
- 2 fresh chopped Mangos
- 1 cup of frozen chopped Mangos*
- 3 frozen quartered Burro Bananas

Cooking instructions
1. Prepare and place all ingredients in the blender.
2. Blend for one minute until smooth.
3. Serve and enjoy your Creamy Mango Smoothie!

Useful Tips
*If you don't have frozen Mango, you can add extra fresh Mango.

Fluffy Avocado Pear Smoothie

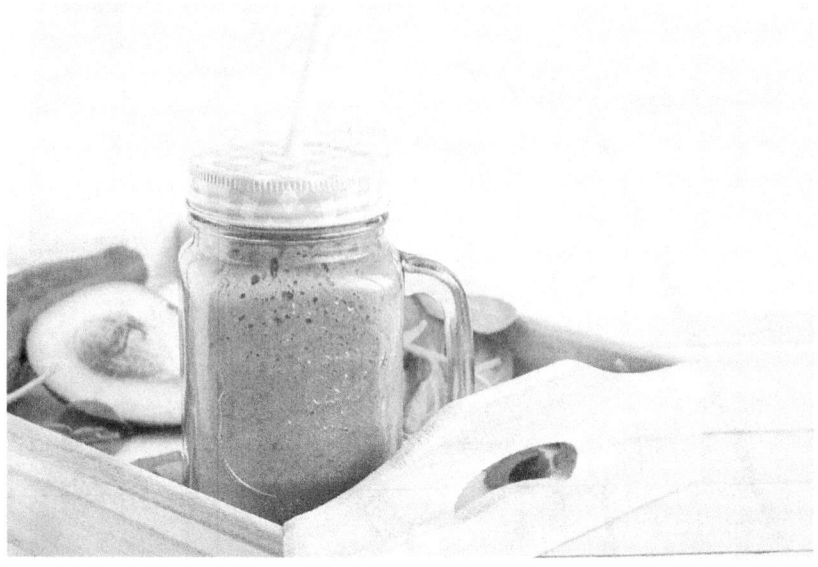

Cooking Time: 10 Minutes

Serving Size: 2 Servings

Ingredients

- 1 cup of cubed Pears*
- 1 cup of chopped Red Apples*
- 1/3 of a medium Avocado
- 2 Medjool Dates
- 1 cup of *Homemade Walnut Milk (see recipe on page 128)***
- 1 tablespoon of Hemp Seeds

- 2 tablespoons of Date Syrup
- 1 handful of Greens *(optional)*
- 1/2 cup of Water
- 1 cup of Ice

Cooking instructions

1. Prepare all ingredients, excluding Ice, and add them to a blender.
2. Blend until smooth.
3. Add Ice and blend once more.
4. Enjoy your Fluffy Avocado Pear Smoothie!

Useful Tips

*Peel and core Pears and Apples before using them.

**If you don't have *Homemade Walnut Milk*, you can substitute *Homemade Hempseed Milk (see recipe on page 132)*.

Apple Pie Smoothie

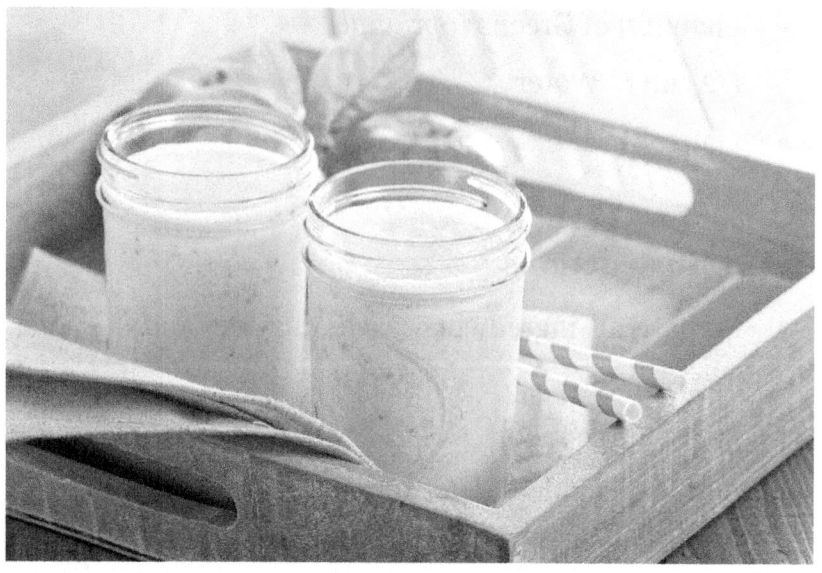

Cooking Time: 5 Minutes

Serving Size: 2 Servings

Ingredients

- 2 cups of fresh Apple Juice
- 1 tablespoon of Sea Moss Gel *(check information on page 18)*
- 1 pinch of Clove Powder
- 1 tablespoon of Ginger *(optional)*
- 2 cups of Ice

Cooking instructions

1. Prepare and place all ingredients into the blender.
2. Blend for one minute until smooth.
3. Add Ice and blend it repeatedly.
4. Enjoy your Apple Pie Smoothie!

Morning Energizer Smoothie

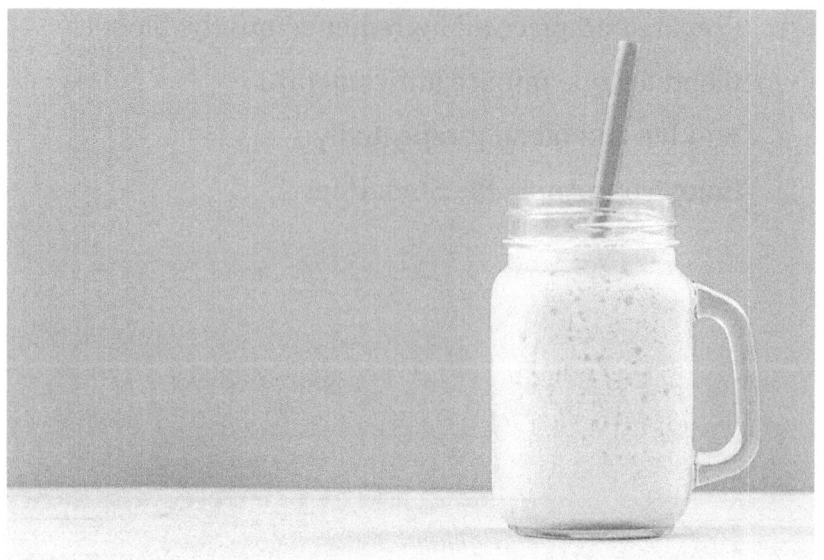

Cooking Time: 20 Minutes

Serving Size: 1 Person

Ingredients

- 1 cup of cubed Melon or Papaya
- 1/2 cup of cooked Amaranth or Quinoa
- 1 cup of *Homemade Walnut Milk (see recipe on page 128)*
- 1 tablespoon of Date Sugar or 1 Date
- 1 teaspoon of Bromide Plus Powder

Cooking instructions

1. Prepare all ingredients and add them to your blender.
2. Blend until it becomes smooth and frothy.
3. Serve it and enjoy your Morning Energizer Smoothie!

Useful Tips

*If you don't have *Homemade Walnut Milk*, you can substitute *Homemade Hempseed Milk (see recipe on page 132)*.

Sunshine Smoothie

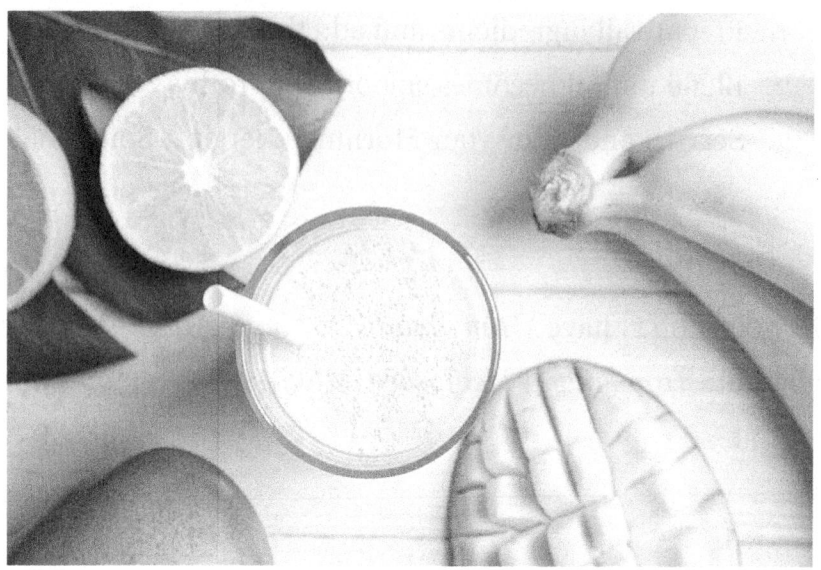

Cooking Time: 10 Minutes

Serving Size: 2 Servings

Ingredients

- 1 chopped Seville Orange
- 1 cup of diced Mango
- 1 cup of Raspberries*
- 1/2 chopped Burro Banana or 1 Baby Banana
- 1 cup of Water

Cooking instructions

1. Combine all ingredients into the blender.
2. Blend until smooth.
3. Serve and enjoy your Sunshine Smoothie!

Useful Tips

*If you don't have fresh berries, you can use frozen ones.

Green Detox Smoothie

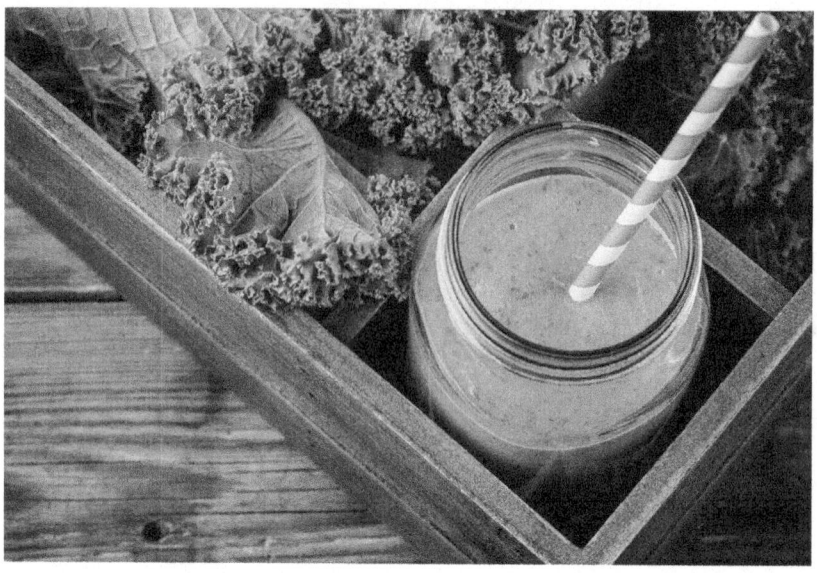

Cooking Time: 10 Minutes

Serving Size: 2 Servings

Ingredients

- 1 cubed Apple*
- 1 cup of chopped Cucumbers
- 2 handfuls of Kale
- 1/4 cup of Lime Juice
- 1 thumb of chopped Ginger *(optional)*
- 1 tablespoon of Sea Moss Gel *(check information on page 18)*
- 2 cups of Coconut Water**

Cooking instructions

1. Prepare all ingredients and add them to your blender.
2. Mix it until it becomes smooth and frothy.
3. Serve it and enjoy your Detox Smoothie!

Useful Tips

*Peel and core Apples before using them.

**If you don't have Coconut Water, you can substitute Spring Water.

Use this smoothie within three days. Store in a glass jar in the refrigerator.

Vegan Detox Smoothie

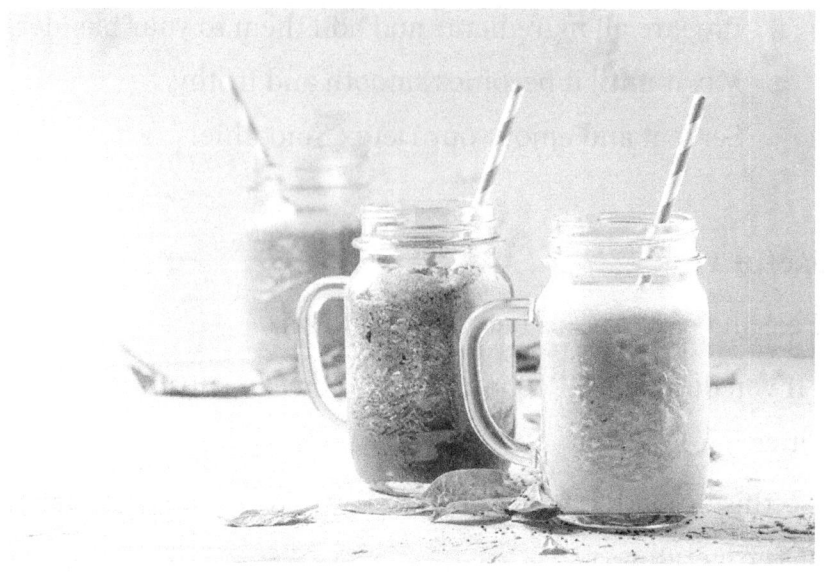

Cooking Time: 10 Minutes

Serving Size: 2 Servings

Ingredients

- 1/2 cup of Blueberries*
- 1 small bunch of Watercress
- 6 medium Dates
- 1 large bunch of Dandelion Greens
- 3 chopped Baby Bananas
- 1 thumb of chopped Ginger *(optional)*
- 1 tablespoon of Burdock Root Powder

- 2 cups of Coconut Water**
- 1/4 cup of Lime Juice

Cooking instructions

1. Prepare and place all ingredients into the blender.
2. Blend for two minutes until smooth.
3. Serve it and enjoy your Vegan Detox Smoothie!

Useful Tips

*If you don't have fresh berries, you can use frozen ones.

**If you don't have Coconut Water, you can substitute Spring Water.

Use this smoothie within three days. Store in a glass jar in the refrigerator.

Mixed Berry Smoothie

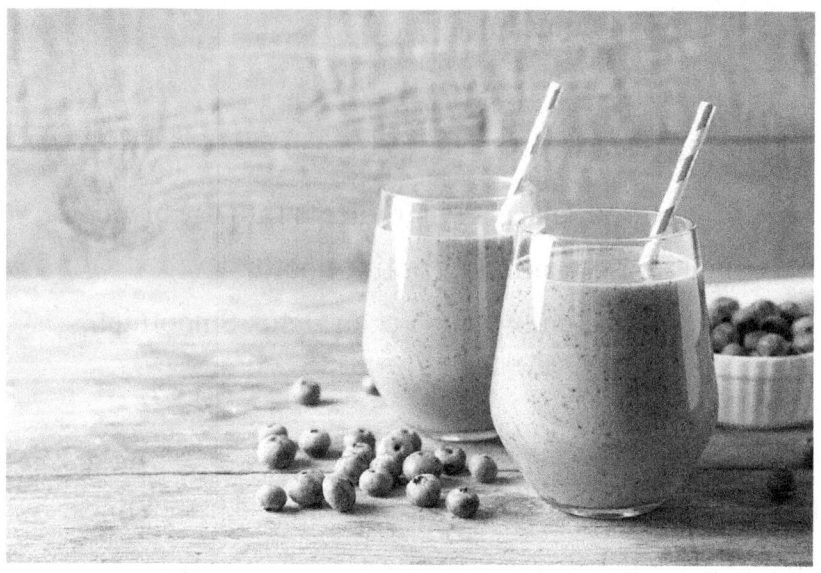

Cooking Time: 5 Minutes

Serving Size: 2 Servings

Ingredients

- 2 handfuls of Strawberries*
- 2 handfuls of Blueberries*
- 2 Burro Bananas
- 2 cups of *Homemade Walnut Milk (see recipe on page 128)***
- 1 cup of Water

Cooking instructions

1. Prepare all ingredients and add them to your blender.
2. Blend until it becomes smooth and frothy.
3. Serve it and enjoy your Mixed Berry Smoothie!

Useful Tips

*If you don't have fresh berries or bananas, you can use frozen ones.

**If you don't have *Homemade Walnut Milk*, you can substitute *Homemade Hempseed Milk (see recipe on page 132)*.

Hydrating Recovery Smoothie

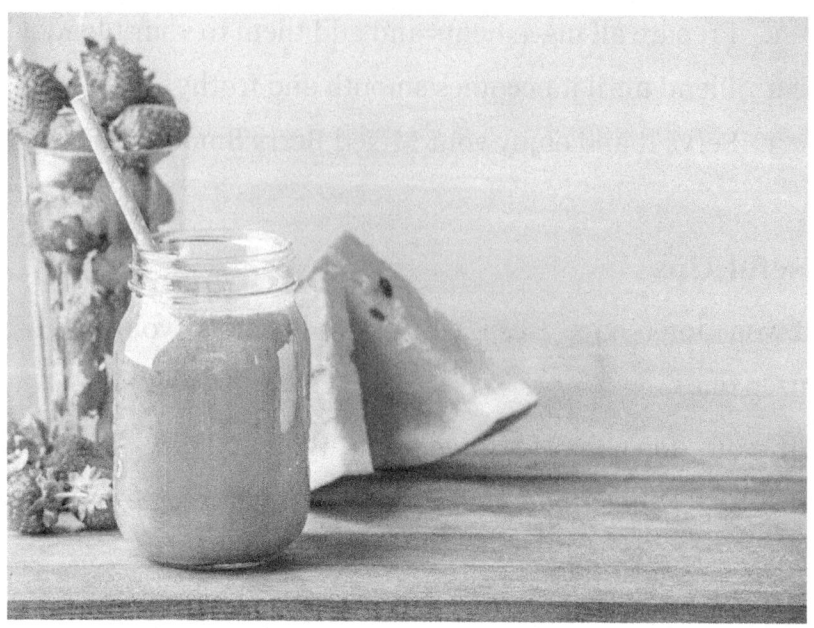

Cooking Time: 5 Minutes

Serving Size: 1 Serving

Ingredients

- 1 cup of Watermelon chunks
- 1 cup of Strawberries*
- 1 tablespoon of Date Syrup
- 1 cup of Coconut Water**

Cooking instructions

1. Combine all ingredients in the blender.
2. Blend until smooth.
3. Serve and enjoy your Hydrating Recovery Smoothie!

Useful Tips

*If you don't have fresh berries, you can use frozen ones.

**If you don't have Coconut Milk, you can substitute *Homemade Walnut Milk (see recipe on page 128).*

Immune Booster Smoothie

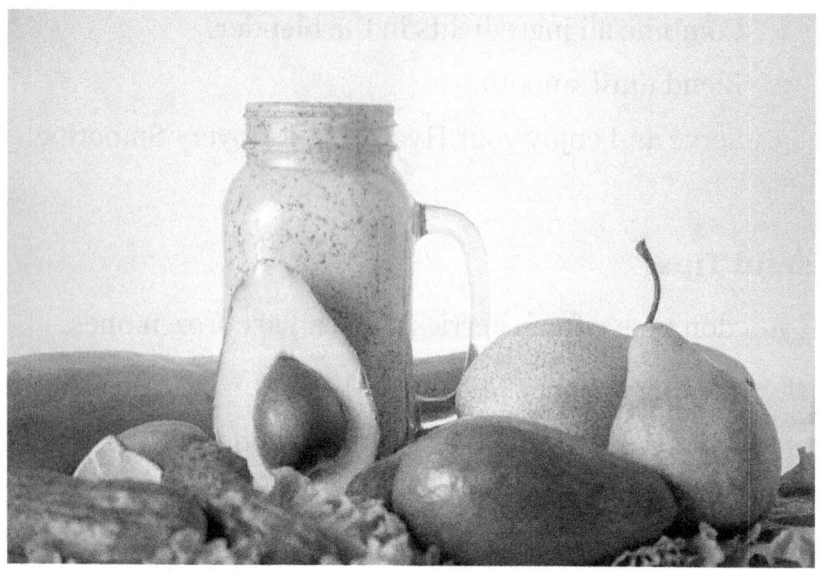

Cooking Time: 10 Minutes

Serving Size: 1 Serving

Ingredients

- 1/4 Avocado
- 1 chopped Pear*
- 1/2 chopped Cucumber
- 1 handful of Romaine Lettuce
- Date Sugar *(optional)*
- 1 handful of Watercress
- 1/2 cup of Spring Water

Cooking instructions

1. Prepare and place all ingredients in the blender.
2. Blend for one minute until smooth.
3. Enjoy your Immune Booster Smoothie!

Useful Tips

*Peel and core Pears before using them.

Sweet and Tart Smoothie

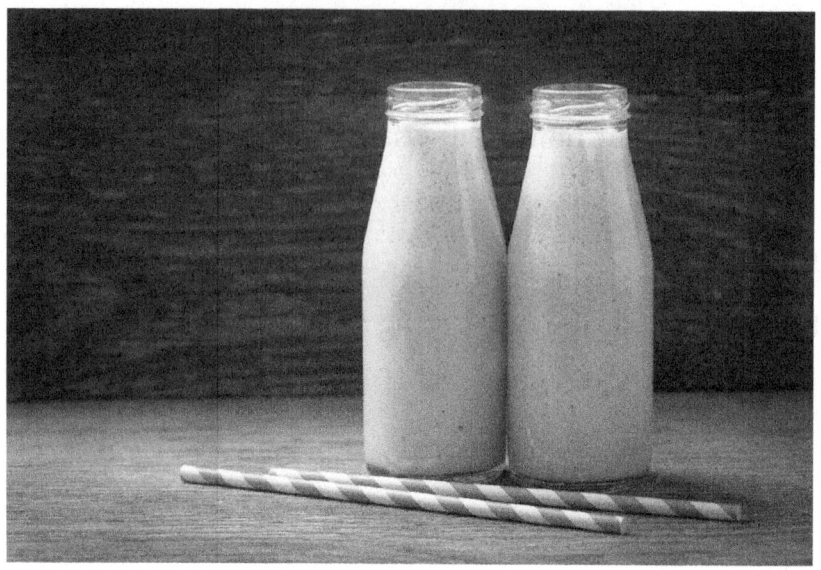

Cooking Time: 5 Minutes

Serving Size: 1 Serving

Ingredients

- 1/2 cup of Red Currants
- 2 quartered Peaches
- 1 tablespoon of Agave Syrup
- 1 teaspoon of Bromide Plus Powder
- 1 cup of Coconut Milk*
- 1/2 cup of Ice

Cooking instructions

1. Prepare all ingredients except Ice and add them to a blender.
2. Blend until smooth.
3. Add Ice and blend once more.
4. Enjoy your Sweet and Tart Smoothie!

Useful Tips

*If you don't have Coconut Milk, you can substitute Spring Water or *Homemade Walnut Milk (see recipe on page 128).*

Berry Peach Smoothie

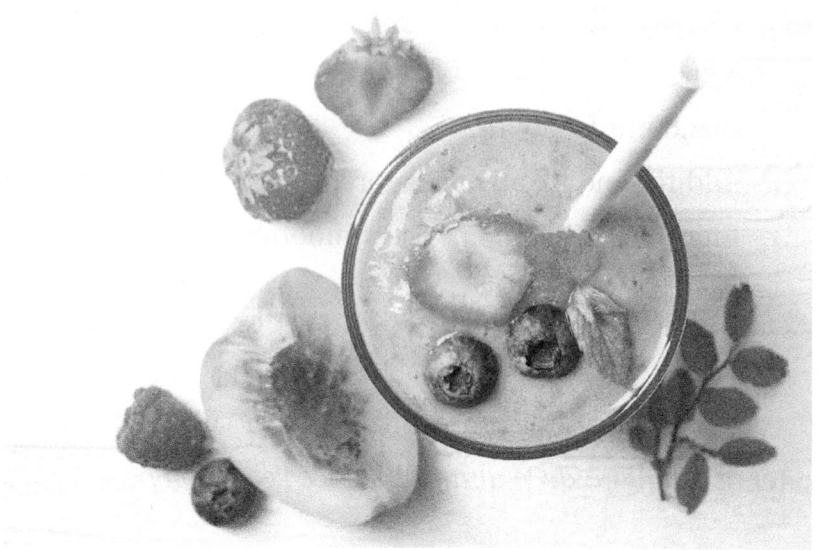

Cooking Time: 10 Minutes

Serving Size: 1 Serving

Ingredients

- 1/2 cup of Cherries
- 1/2 cup of Strawberries*
- 1/2 cup of quartered Peaches
- 1/2 cup of Blueberries*
- 1 tablespoon of Sea Moss Gel *(check information on page 18)*
- 1 tablespoon of Agave Syrup

- 1 cup of Coconut Milk**
- 1 tablespoon of Hemp Seeds

Cooking instructions

1. Prepare all ingredients and add them to your blender.
2. Mix until it becomes smooth and frothy.
3. Serve it and enjoy your Berry Peach Smoothie!

Useful Tips

*If you don't have fresh berries, you can use frozen ones.

**If you don't have Coconut Milk, you can substitute Spring Water.

Add extra 1/4 cup of Coconut Milk or Spring Water if the smoothie is too thick.

CONCLUSION

Congratulations!

Now you have learned 77 simple, Doctor Sebi alkaline diet recipes. That means you can surprise yourself, your family, and your friends with new, delicious dishes, snacks, salads, desserts, or smoothies.

Not only will you be eating tasty meals, you will also be helping yourself and your family to feel better and improve overall health just by eating approved Doctor Sebi food. How great is that?

Now there is just one thing for you to do: Take action!

I know, you have most likely been in this position before. Maybe you have already tried other diets in the past, but you just can't find a suitable nutritional plan for you.

This time will be different. I promise!

Take care of yourself and live a long, healthy life!

Thank you for buying!

Made in the USA
Las Vegas, NV
17 June 2023

73563431R00115